Anesthesia

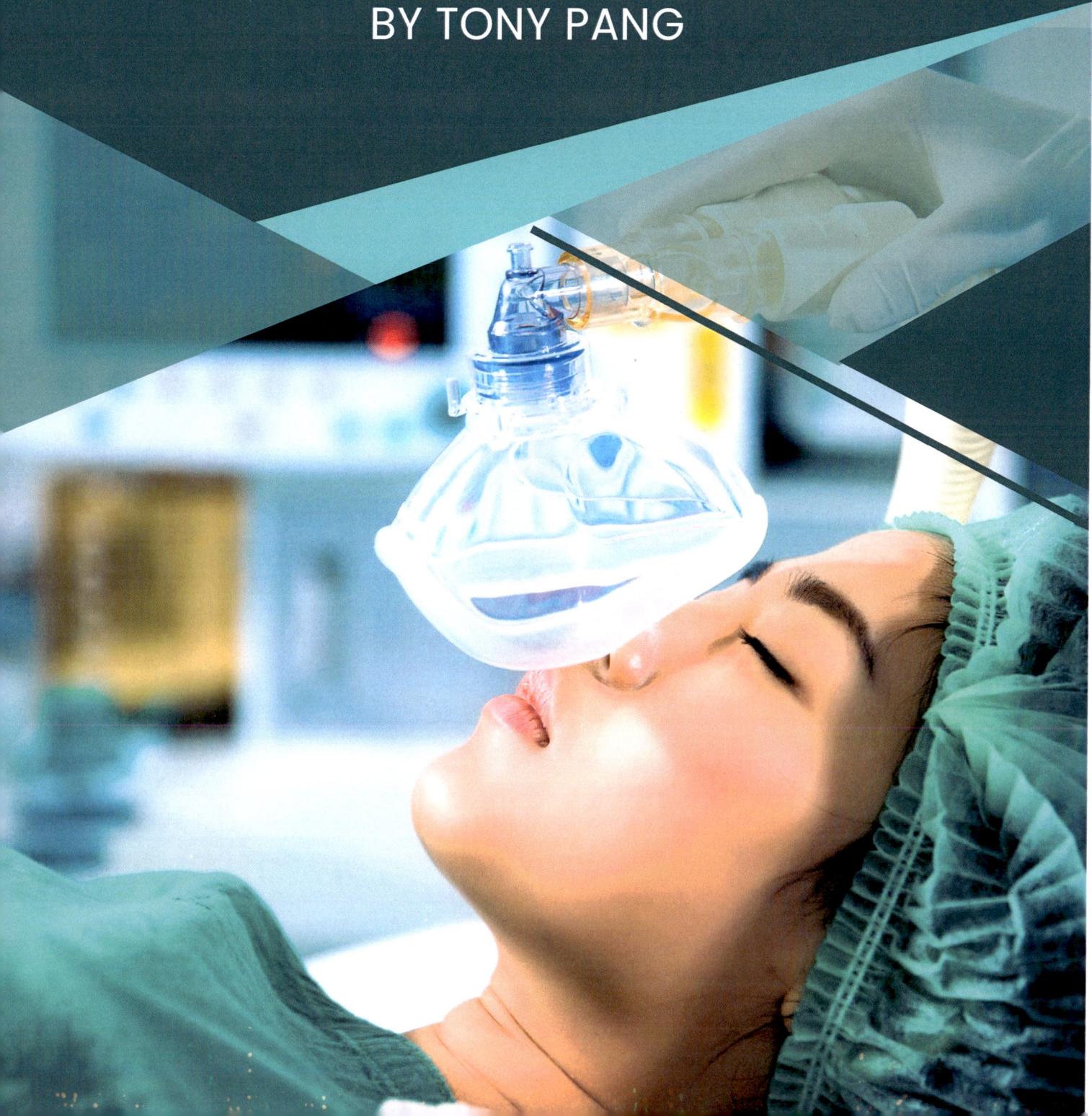

TECHNICIAN SURVIVAL GUIDE

ANESTHESIA EQUIPMENT:

BY TONY PANG

DEDICATION

Mama, this is for you. Thank you for constantly being there for me, and thank you for the beanpies.

PREFACE

As the chief technician at Strong Memorial Hospital, one of my responsibilities was to supervise the preparation of all our anesthesia technicians. I saw there was a great deal of data to process and remember as an anesthesia tech. I also found that everyone was at different levels in their training. I said to myself, "I wish there was a smaller companion book to go along with our large anesthesia training manual to help our techs as they proceed in their training." Of course, there wasn't one, so I decided to write one, with the help of my good friend, RN Patrick Furbert. With the completion of that project, I went on to develop a smaller, less detailed anesthesia technician survival guide that anesthesia technicians all over the world can use.

The purpose of this anesthesia technician survival guide is to support the anesthesia technician as they continue their education and to help them better perform their duties in the operating room environment.

This book is intended to be a guide and not to supersede their hospital individual training, policy, procedures or protocols.

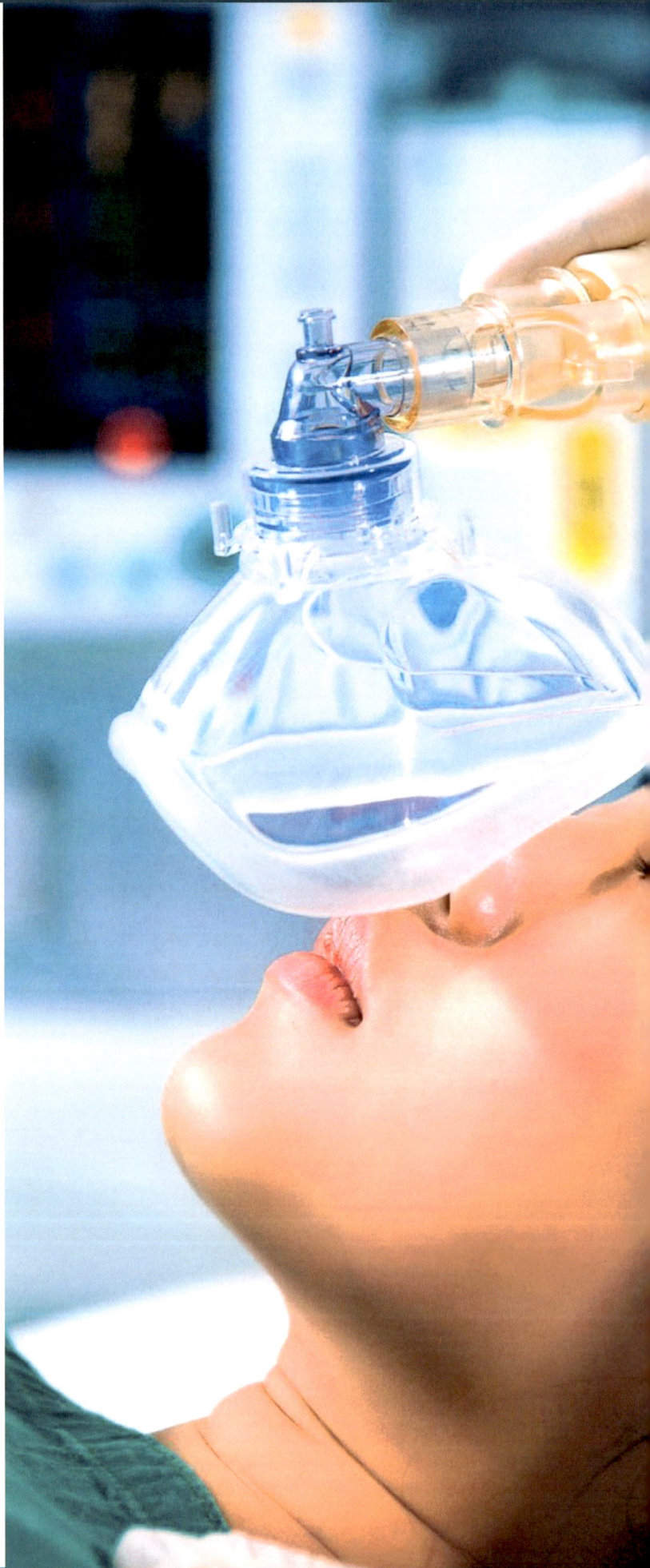

ACKNOWLEDGEMENTS

I would like to acknowledge the anesthesia department at the University of Rochester Medical Center for everything you have done for me. Thanks to Oakwood Hospital for all your patience and support.

Thank you, Elsa Pang. I could not have done this without you. To Erskine Ford, my best friend and writing inspiration. A big thank you to Dr. Liz Elliot. Thank you a million, Ed Griffin, my writing instructor and friend. Thank you, Meredith Egan, Katherine Aubrey, Bea Rhodes, Heartspeak Productions, Evelyn Zellers, Jane Miller, Simon Fraser, and the Center for Restorative Justice at Simon Fraser University.

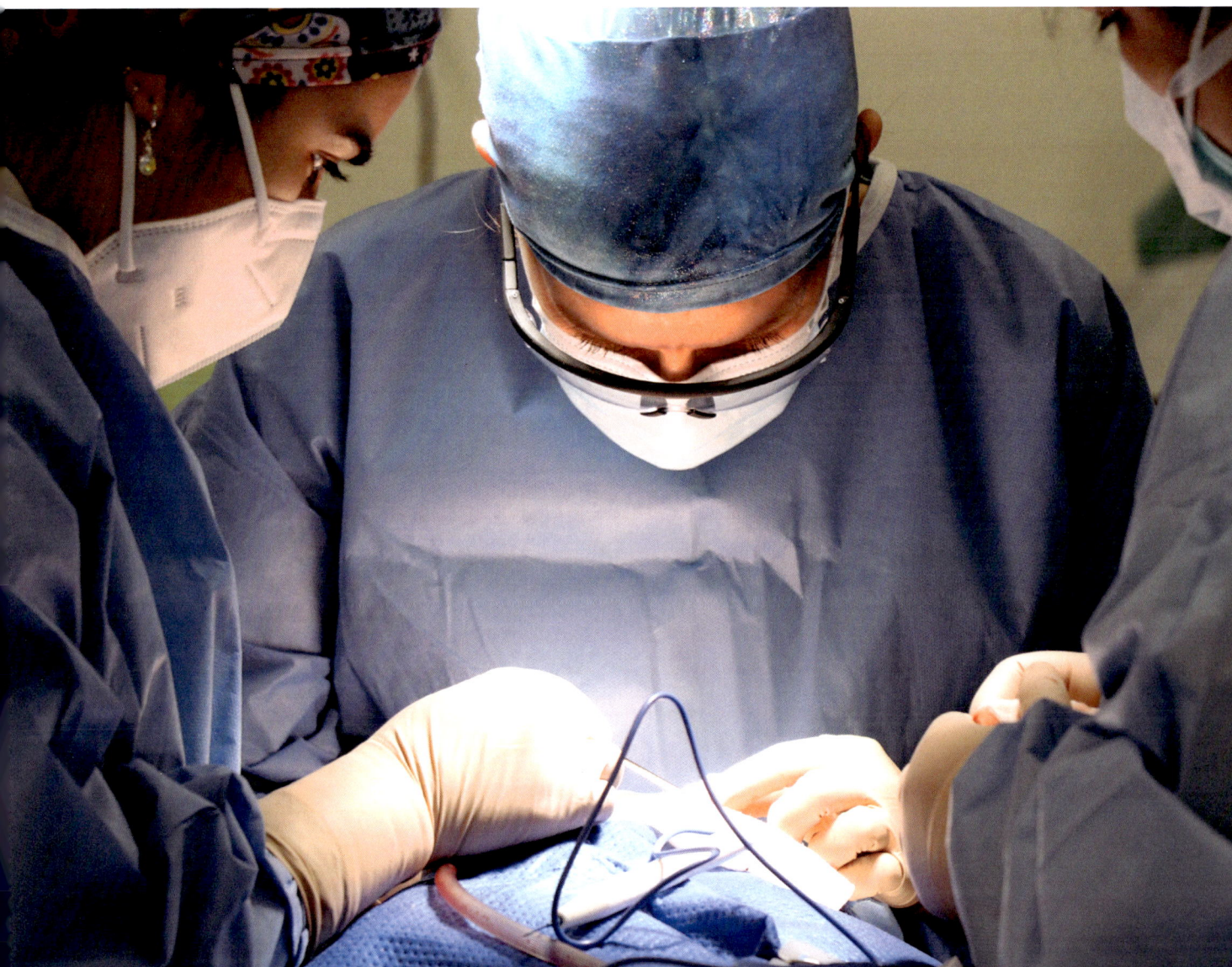

CONTENTS

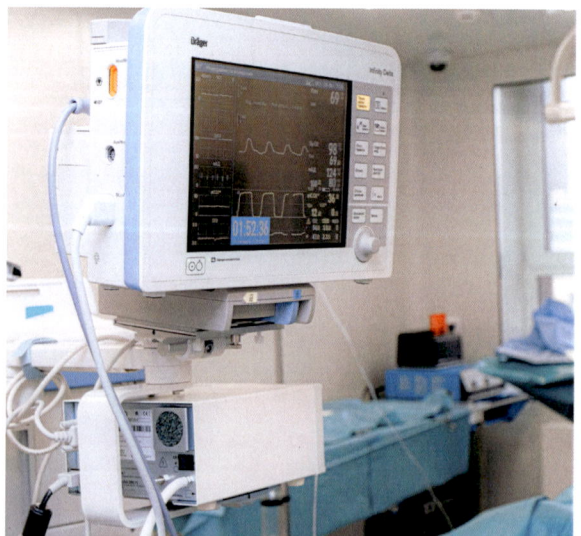

Chapter 1: Introduction to Anesthesia Equipment

1.1 The Role and Importance of Anesthesia Equipment

Anesthesia equipment plays a vital role in the surgical process. It aids the anesthesia provider in safely inducing, maintaining, and reversing the state of anesthesia while monitoring and controlling the patient's vital functions. An Anesthesia Technologist, on the other hand, plays a key role in maintaining, preparing, and troubleshooting the anesthesia equipment.

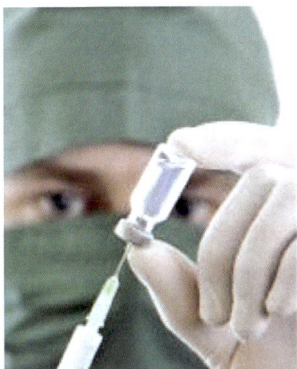

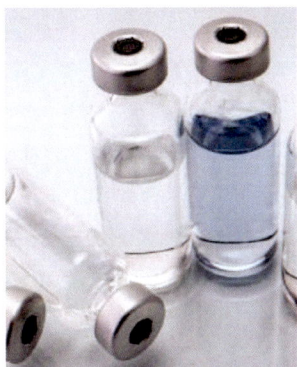

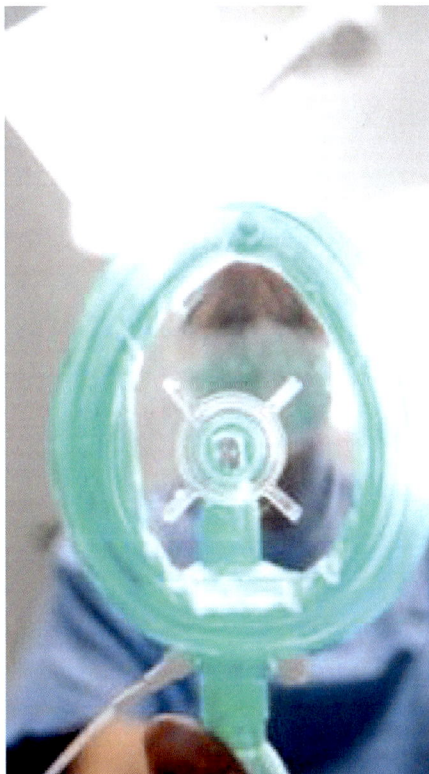

1.2 Types of Anesthesia Equipment

Anesthesia equipment can be broadly categorized into the following types:

Anesthesia Machines: These are used to deliver a precise amount of anesthetic gases and oxygen to the patient.

Airway Equipment: This includes equipment like laryngoscopes, endotracheal tubes, and face masks, used to ensure open and protected airways during anesthesia.

Monitoring Equipment: This includes electrocardiogram machines, blood pressure monitors, and pulse oximeters, among others, to monitor the patient's vital signs throughout the procedure.

IV and Invasive Line Equipment: These devices administer fluids, medications, and measure certain physiological variables.

Waste Gas Scavenging Systems: These systems protect operating room staff from potential anesthetic gas exposure.

1.3 Basic Principles of Operation

Understanding the basic principles of operation of the anesthesia equipment is essential for both the Anesthesia Provider and the Anesthesia Technologist. Here's how the responsibilities could be divided for this section:

DUTIES OF THE ANESTHESIA TECHNOLOGIST:

Step 1: Familiarization with Equipment The technologist should familiarize themselves with the different types of anesthesia equipment, including their components and operation. They should be able to identify all components of the anesthesia machine, understand the functionality of each, and the sequence of events in the machine's operation.

Step 2: Maintenance and Troubleshooting The technologist should be aware of the regular maintenance schedules of each piece of equipment and carry out the necessary tasks. They should also be trained to troubleshoot common issues that may arise during the setup or operation of the equipment.

DUTIES OF THE ANESTHESIA PROVIDER:

Step 1: Understanding the Principles of Operation The provider should have an indepth understanding of how the anesthesia equipment works. This includes how the anesthetic gases are delivered, how the airway equipment maintains a clear airway, and how the monitors read and display the patient's vital signs.

Step 2: Application to Patient Care The anesthesia provider should understand how the principles of operation apply to patient care. This includes knowing which equipment to use in different scenarios, how to adjust settings based on the patient's status, and how to respond to changes in monitor readings.

This chapter lays the foundation for the rest of the guide, which will delve deeper into the setup, operation, and maintenance of each type of anesthesia equipment. Remember, a successful operation hinges on the seamless operation and handling of the anesthesia equipment by both the Anesthesia Provider and the Anesthesia Technologist.

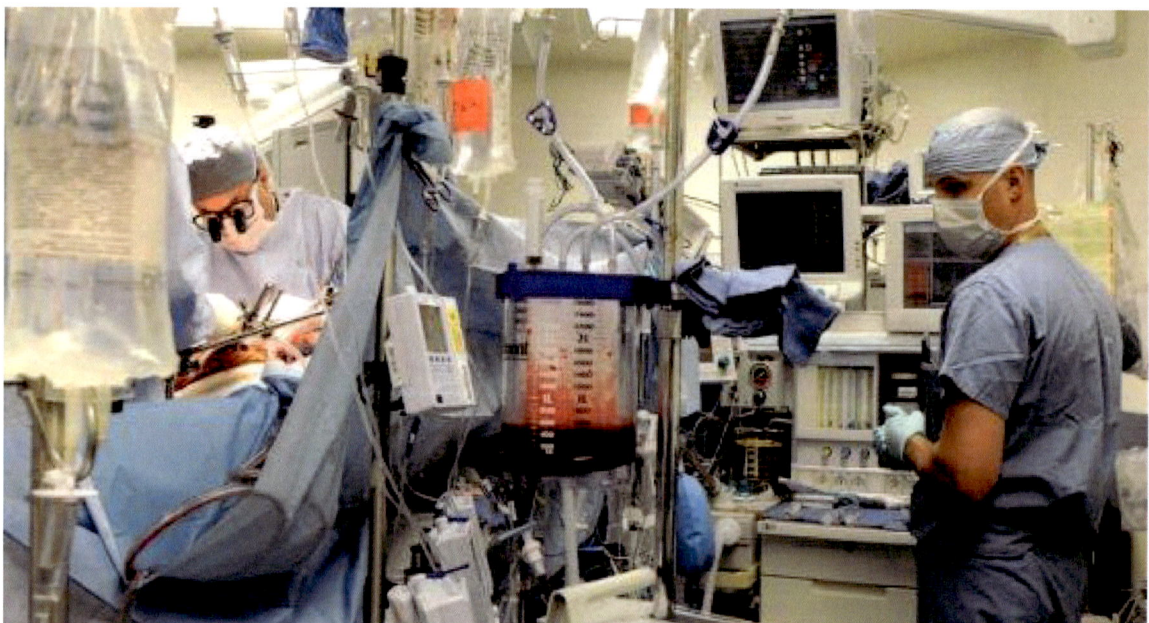

Chapter 2: Setting Up and Operating Anesthesia Machines

2.1 Overview

Anesthesia machines are complex, yet crucial devices that deliver mixed gases (oxygen, air, nitrous oxide) and volatile anesthetics to the patient while allowing for patient ventilation and monitoring. They also contain various safety systems designed to prevent hypoxic gas delivery or excessive pressure delivery to the patient. Understanding their setup and operation is vital for both the Anesthesia Provider and the Anesthesia Technologist.

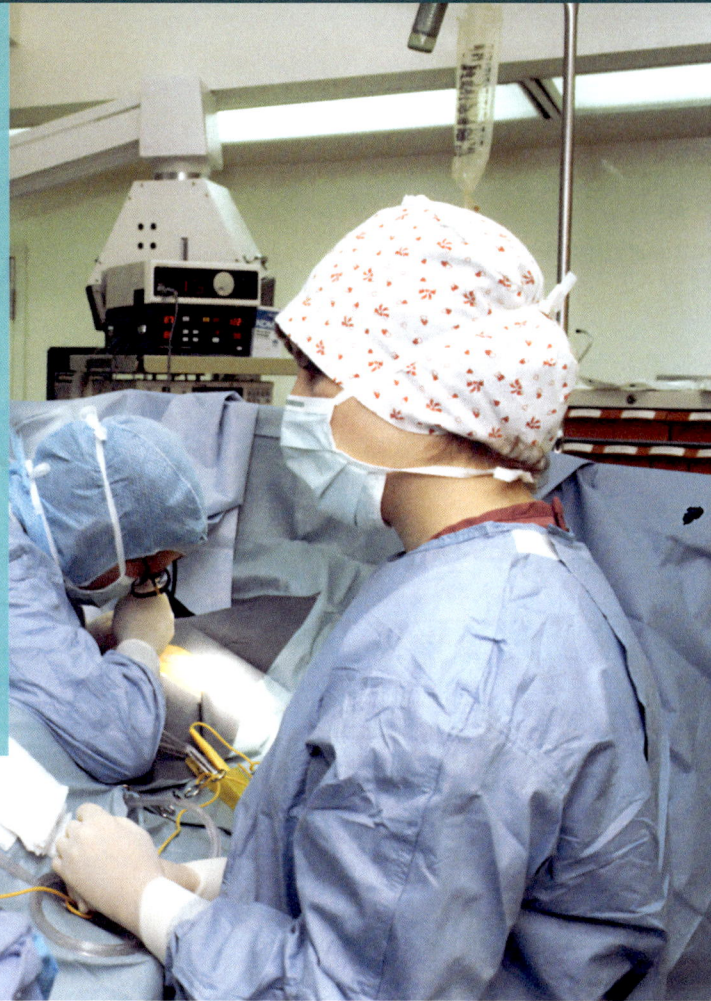

2.2 Components of Anesthesia Machines

Anesthesia machines typically consist of the following components:

- Gas supply and control system (includes pipelines, cylinders, pressure gauges, regulators, flowmeters)
- Anesthetic vaporizer
- Breathing system
- Ventilator
- Monitoring and alarm system
- Scavenging system

2.3 Step-by-Step Setup and Operation

DUTIES OF THE ANESTHESIA TECHNOLOGIST:

Step 1: Gas Supply Setup The technologist should begin by checking the oxygen and nitrous oxide pipeline pressures and cylinder supply. They should ensure all cylinders are properly attached and have adequate pressure.

Step 2: Anesthetic Vaporizer Setup Next, they must attach the anesthetic vaporizer securely and fill it with the selected volatile anesthetic agent, ensuring not to overfill or mix agents.

Step 3: Breathing System Assembly The technologist should then assemble the breathing system, which typically includes a circle system with inspiratory and expiratory valves, carbon dioxide absorber, and breathing bag. All connections should be secure.

Step 4: Initial Checks The technologist should perform initial machine checks. These include checking for leaks in the gas delivery system, ensuring correct function of the pressure relief devices, and verifying the correct function of the breathing system, including the CO_2 absorber and breathing bag.

DUTIES OF THE ANESTHESIA PROVIDER:

Step 5: Final Machine Check The anesthesia provider should perform the final machine check, including checking for correct function of the ventilator, vaporizer, and all alarms. This is also a good time to ensure the availability of a functioning suction device and appropriate airway management equipment.

Step 6: Patient Connection After the patient is anesthetized, the provider must connect the patient to the machine via the endotracheal tube or mask, ensuring a secure and leak-free connection.

Step 7: Monitor Setup and Operation The provider should then set up and initiate the monitors, including ECG, pulse oximeter, non-invasive blood pressure monitor, and capnograph. The provider should understand how to interpret these monitor readings and adjust the anesthetic delivery accordingly.

Step 8: Anesthesia Delivery The provider will manage the delivery of anesthesia by adjusting the gas flows and vaporizer setting, monitoring the patient's depth of anesthesia, and making necessary adjustments. This includes understanding how to operate the ventilator if necessary, and adjusting settings based on the patient's needs.

Step 9: Emergence At the end of the procedure, the provider should know how to safely discontinue the delivery of anesthetic agents and facilitate the patient's emergence from anesthesia, including disconnecting the patient from the machine.

Step 10: Post-Operative Machine Check Lastly, the provider should perform a post-operative machine check, including turning off the machine and all gas flows, emptying the breathing bag, and ensuring the vaporizer is off and adequately filled for the next case.

This detailed step-by-step guide should facilitate a deeper understanding of the setup and operation of anesthesia machines. With clearly demarcated responsibilities, the Anesthesia Provider and the Anesthesia Technologist can work seamlessly to ensure patient safety and comfort throughout the perioperative period.

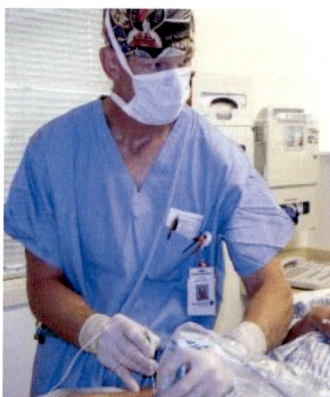

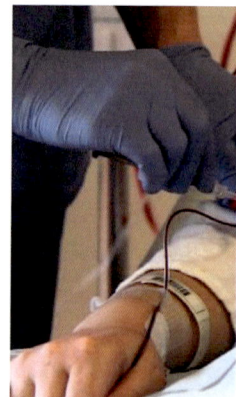

Chapter 3: Anesthesia Delivery Systems and Ventilators

In this chapter, we will delve into the intricacies of anesthesia delivery systems
and the role of ventilators in the delivery of anesthesia. We will explore the various types of anesthesia delivery systems, discuss the importance of ventilators in anesthesia practice, and provide detailed instructions on the operation and setup of ventilators.

3.1 Types of Anesthesia Delivery Systems

Anesthesia delivery systems are designed to deliver anesthetic agents, oxygen, and other gases to the patient while ensuring their safety and comfort. There are several types of anesthesia delivery systems commonly used:

Open Circuit Systems: Open circuit systems, such as the Ayre's T-piece and the Bain system, allow fresh gas flow to pass through the system and directly exit into the atmosphere. These systems are primarily used for low-flow anesthesia, where a minimal amount of fresh gas flow is required.

Semi-Closed Circuit Systems: Semi-closed circuit systems, including the Circle system and the Mapleson systems (A to E), incorporate a breathing circuit that allows for the rebreathing of exhaled gases with the addition of fresh gases. Carbon dioxide is removed from the system using carbon dioxide absorbers. These systems are commonly used for general anesthesia and provide more efficient use of anesthetic gases.

Closed Circuit Systems: Closed circuit systems, such as the Circle system with a CO_2 absorber and the Jackson-Rees modification, enable the complete recycling of exhaled gases by removing carbon dioxide and replenishing oxygen. Closed circuit systems are used for low-flow or minimal-flow anesthesia and conserve anesthetic gases while maintaining a closed-loop system.

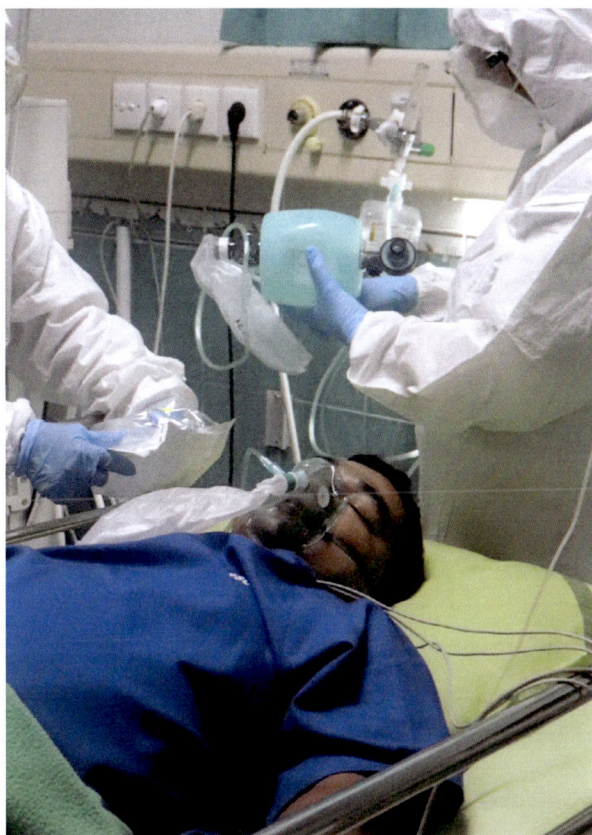

Total Intravenous Anesthesia (TIVA) Systems: TIVA systems involve the administration of intravenous anesthetic agents without the use of inhaled gases. These systems often utilize a target-controlled infusion (TCI) pump to deliver precise and controlled amounts of intravenous anesthetics.

The Anesthesia Provider is responsible for selecting the appropriate anesthesia delivery system based on the patient's needs, the type of surgery or procedure, and other factors. They should be knowledgeable about the different systems and their advantages and limitations to ensure the safe and effective administration of anesthesia.

ANESTHESIA TECHNOLOGIST'S ROLE:

Assisting the Anesthesia Provider in setting up and preparing the anesthesia delivery system, ensuring all components are present and functioning properly.

Checking the anesthesia machine for leaks, proper gas supply, and functioning of monitors and alarms.

Assisting in assembling the breathing circuit, ensuring proper connections and functionality.

Collaborating with the Anesthesia Provider to confirm the appropriate anesthesia delivery system based on patient and procedural requirements.

Assisting in monitoring the patient during anesthesia, including observing the breathing circuit and adjusting components as needed.

3.2 The Role of Ventilators in Anesthesia Delivery

Ventilators play a vital role in anesthesia delivery by providing controlled and regulated mechanical ventilation to patients under anesthesia. They ensure adequate oxygenation and carbon dioxide removal, support respiratory function, and maintain optimal lung mechanics. Ventilators are particularly important during general anesthesia, as they assist with the exchange of respiratory gases and help manage the patient's airway.

The Anesthesia Provider is responsible for selecting and operating the appropriate ventilator mode and settings based on the patient's condition, the type of surgery or procedure, and the desired respiratory goals. They must be knowledgeable about the different modes and parameters available on the ventilator and understand how to optimize ventilation and oxygenation.

ANESTHESIA TECHNOLOGIST'S ROLE:

Assisting the Anesthesia Provider in preparing and setting up the ventilator, ensuring all necessary connections, tubing, and filters are in place.

Collaborating with the Anesthesia Provider to verify the appropriate ventilator mode and settings based on patient and procedural requirements.

Assisting in placing and securing the patient's endotracheal tube or other airway devices as directed by the Anesthesia Provider.

Monitoring the ventilator for proper function, including alarm settings, tidal volume, respiratory rate, and oxygen concentration.

Assisting in troubleshooting ventilator alarms or malfunctions, notifying the Anesthesia Provider or biomedical engineering as needed.

3.3 Operation and Setup of Ventilators

Operating and setting up ventilators require a thorough understanding of the specific model and its features. Here are some general steps to consider:

Preparation: Ensure the ventilator is clean, calibrated, and functioning properly. Check the gas supply, power source, and connections to the anesthesia machine. Verify the availability of necessary accessories, such as breathing circuits, humidifiers, and filters.

Patient Preparation: Prepare the patient for mechanical ventilation, which may involve intubation, placement of a supraglottic airway, or other airway management techniques. Confirm proper positioning of the patient, secure the airway device, and ensure adequate monitoring of the patient's vital signs.

Ventilator Setup: Power on the ventilator and select the appropriate ventilation mode based on the patient's condition and procedure. Set the desired parameters, including tidal volume, respiratory rate, positive end-expiratory pressure (PEEP), and inspired oxygen concentration (FiO2).

Monitoring: Continuously monitor the patient's vital signs, including oxygen saturation, end-tidal carbon dioxide (EtCO2), and airway pressures. Ensure that alarms are properly set and functional to alert you of any deviations from the set parameters.

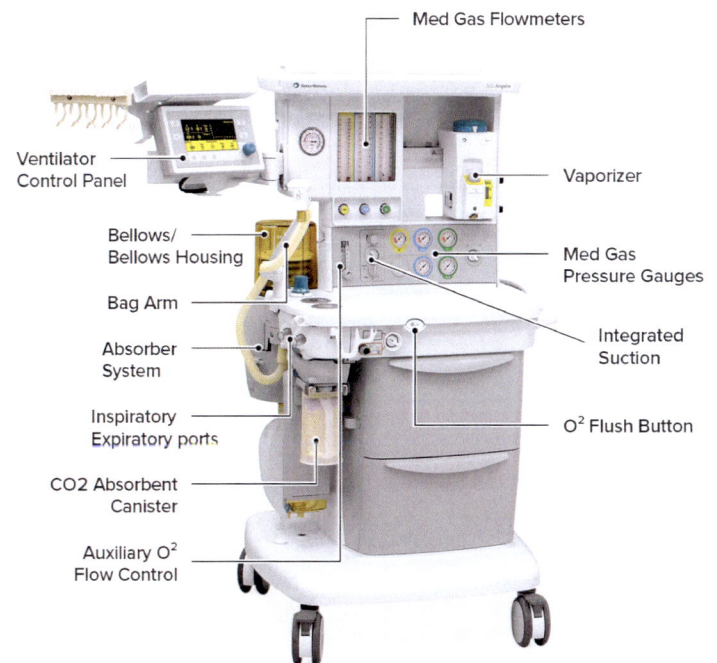

GE Aespire Components and Controls

Initiation of Mechanical Ventilation: Initiate mechanical ventilation by connecting the patient's airway device to the ventilator circuit. Confirm proper placement and secure the connections. Start the ventilator and observe the patient's response to mechanical ventilation.

Adjustments: Monitor the patient's response to mechanical ventilation and make necessary adjustments to the ventilator settings. This may include modifying tidal volume, respiratory rate, PEEP, FiO2, or switching to different ventilation modes to optimize ventilation and oxygenation.

Alarm Management: Continuously monitor the ventilator alarms and respond promptly to any alarms or deviations from the set parameters. Troubleshoot alarm issues and make appropriate adjustments to ensure patient safety.

Documentation: Document all relevant information related to the ventilator setup, parameters, adjustments, and patient responses. This includes recording ventilator settings, patient monitoring data, and any interventions performed.

ANESTHESIA PROVIDER'S ROLE:

Selecting the appropriate ventilation mode and settings based on the patient's condition, surgical procedure, and respiratory goals.

Monitoring the patient's response to mechanical ventilation, including lung compliance, oxygenation, and ventilation parameters.

Making necessary adjustments to the ventilator settings to optimize ventilation and maintain patient stability.

Ensuring proper communication with the Anesthesia Technologist and other healthcare professionals regarding any ventilator-related concerns or changes in patient status.

ANESTHESIA TECHNOLOGIST'S ROLE:

Assisting in the setup and preparation of the ventilator, ensuring all connections, tubing, and filters are properly assembled.

Monitoring the ventilator for proper function, including alarm settings, tidal volume, respiratory rate, PEEP, and FiO2.

Assisting in troubleshooting ventilator alarms or malfunctions, notifying the Anesthesia Provider or biomedical engineering as needed.

Collaborating with the Anesthesia Provider to provide support during airway management, securing the airway device, and ensuring adequate ventilation.

By following the proper setup and operation procedures for anesthesia delivery systems and ventilators, anesthesia professionals can ensure safe and effective delivery of anesthesia, optimize patient outcomes, and maintain patient safety throughout the perioperative period. It is crucial to adhere to institutional policies, manufacturer guidelines, and industry best practices to provide the highest standard of care.

Chapter 4: Mastery of Anesthesia Delivery Systems: Setup, Operation, and Maintenance

4.1 Introduction

An anesthesia delivery system (ADS) is the central hub of an operating room, responsible for the safe and effective delivery of inhalational and intravenous anesthetics to patients. This chapter provides a detailed step-by-step guide on setting up and operating an ADS, with roles specified for the Anesthesia Provider and Anesthesia Technologist.

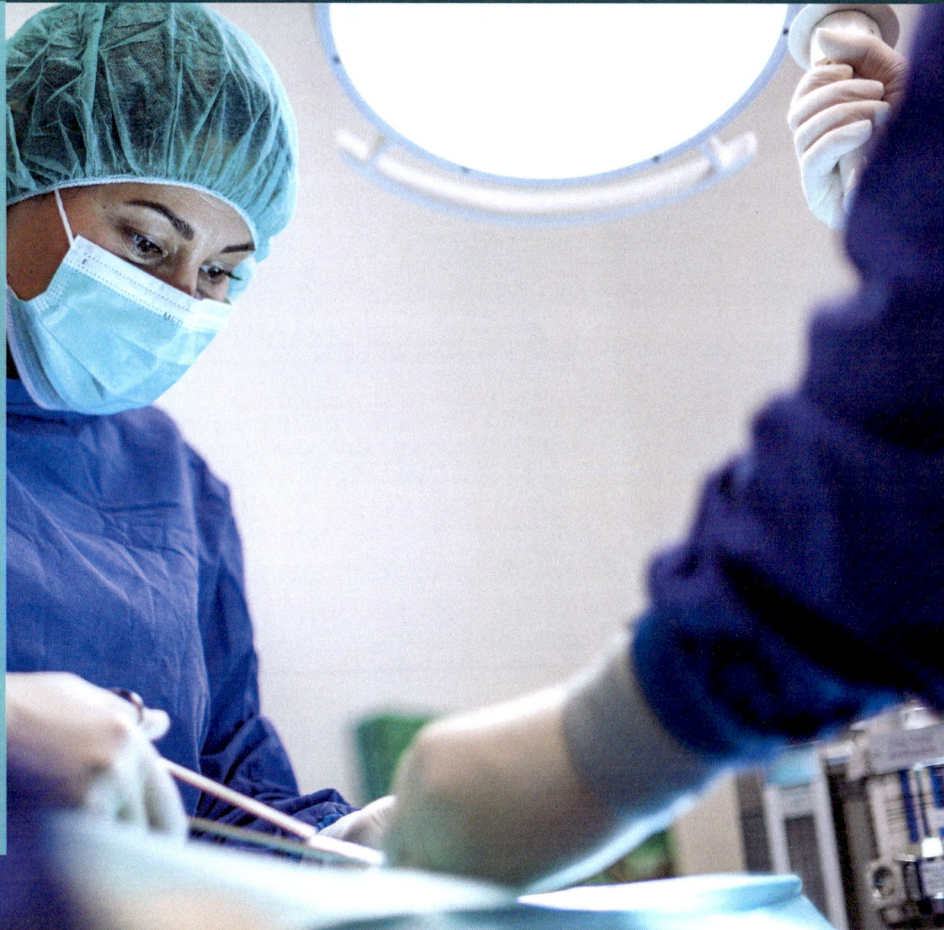

4.2 Key Components of an Anesthesia Delivery System

The ADS consists of several essential components:

- **Gas Supply:** This includes the central pipeline supply and backup cylinder supply for oxygen, nitrous oxide, and air.
- **Anesthetic Vaporizer:** Used to deliver inhalational anesthetic agents.
- **Ventilator:** Provides mechanical ventilation to the patient.
- Breathing Circuit: Connects the patient to the ADS and includes the inspiratory and expiratory limbs, along with CO_2 absorbent canisters.
- **Intravenous Infusion Pumps:** For the delivery of intravenous anesthetics and other drugs.
- **Patient Monitors:** As discussed in Chapter 3, monitors for ECG, SpO2, NIBP, EtCO2, BIS, temperature, and nerve stimulation.

4.3 Step-by-Step Setup and Operation

DUTIES OF THE ANESTHESIA TECHNOLOGIST:

Step 1: ADS Preparation Ensure all components of the ADS are in place, clean, and functional. Ensure backup cylinders are filled, and all alarms on the ADS are functional.
Step 2: Vaporizer Setup Ensure the correct anesthetic agent is filled in the vaporizer and that it is securely attached to the ADS.
Step 3: Ventilator Preparation Check the functionality of the ventilator, including the proper assembly of the breathing circuit and the CO_2 absorbent level.
Step 4: Intravenous Infusion Pumps Setup Check the functionality of infusion pumps, prepare syringes or infusion bags with the required anesthetics or drugs, and ensure correct labeling.

DUTIES OF THE ANESTHESIA PROVIDER:

Step 5: ADS Operation Before the patient's arrival in the operating room, check the proper functioning of all the components of the ADS, including gas flows, vaporizer settings, ventilator settings, and proper functioning of all alarms.
Step 6: Patient Connection Connect the patient to the ADS once they are positioned and secured on the operating table. This includes connecting the patient to the breathing circuit, starting the delivery of inhalational anesthetics, if required, and starting intravenous infusions.
Step 7: Intraoperative Management Manage the delivery of anesthetics based on the patient's response, the stage of surgery, and monitoring data. Ensure all alarms are active and respond to any alarms promptly.
Step 8: Postoperative Management At the end of the surgery, stop the delivery of anesthetics, disconnect the patient from the ADS, and prepare the patient for transport out of the operating room.
Step 9: ADS Postoperative Check Ensure the ADS is clean and ready for the next use. Refill the vaporizer and CO_2 absorbent, if necessary. Report any equipment malfunctions for immediate repair.

By following these detailed instructions, the Anesthesia Provider and Anesthesia Technologist can ensure safe and efficient use of the Anesthesia Delivery System, improving patient outcomes and workflow in the operating room.

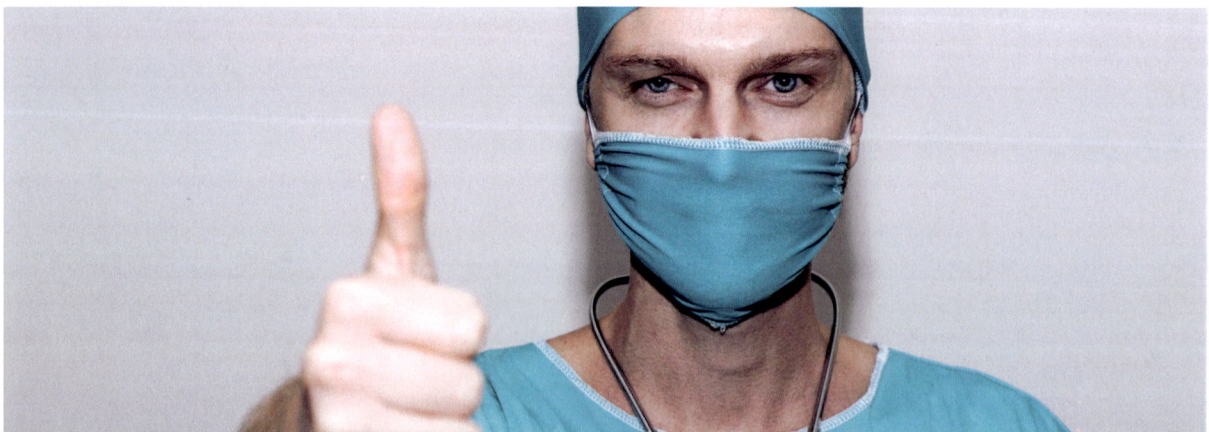

Chapter 5: Ensuring Safety with Anesthesia Monitoring Equipment

5.1 Introduction

Patient monitoring is a critical component of anesthesia delivery. With an array of devices providing real-time data about a patient's physiological state, anesthesia professionals can make timely, informed decisions. Both Anesthesia Providers and Anesthesia Technologists must understand how to set up, operate, and maintain these monitoring devices.

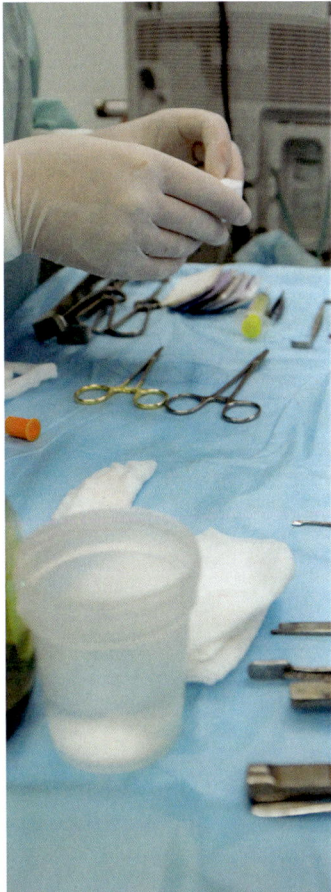

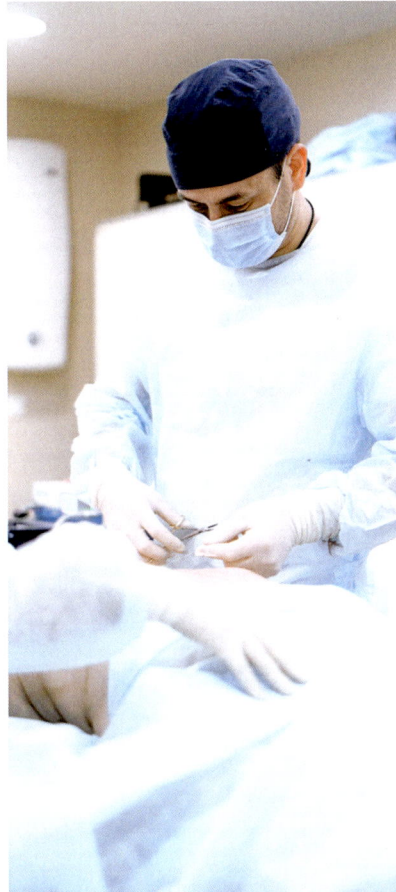

5.2 Essential Anesthesia Monitoring Equipment

Typical monitoring equipment in the operating room includes:

Electrocardiogram (ECG): Monitors heart rate and rhythm.

Pulse Oximeter (SpO2): Measures the oxygen saturation of the patient's blood.

Non-Invasive Blood Pressure Monitor (NIBP): Provides periodic measurements of the patient's blood pressure.

Capnograph (EtCO2): Measures the concentration of carbon dioxide in exhaled breath, which reflects ventilatory status.

Bispectral Index Monitor (BIS): A tool to assess the depth of anesthesia.

Temperature monitor: Helps to avoid hypothermia or hyperthermia.

Nerve stimulator: Used to monitor neuromuscular blockade in patients given muscle relaxants.

5.3 Step-by-Step Setup and Operation

DUTIES OF THE ANESTHESIA TECHNOLOGIST:

Step 1: Equipment Preparation The technologist should ensure all monitoring devices are available, functional, and clean. They should also prepare necessary accessories, like ECG leads, SpO2 sensors, blood pressure cuffs, temperature probes, and capnography sampling lines.

Step 2: Initial Setup The technologist should connect all monitors to the anesthesia machine or standalone monitor as applicable, ensuring all cables and connections are secure and functional. They should perform a self-test if available.

Step 3: Calibration The technologist should calibrate the monitors as required. For example, zeroing the NIBP, or performing a pre-use check on the capnograph.

DUTIES OF THE ANESTHESIA PROVIDER:

Step 4: Patient Connection The anesthesia provider should attach the ECG leads, SpO2 sensor, and blood pressure cuff to the patient. They should insert the temperature probe in an appropriate location (e.g., nasopharynx, esophagus, bladder) and attach the capnography sampling line to the breathing circuit.

Step 5: Monitor Operation The anesthesia provider should then activate each monitor, ensuring that each is providing accurate data. The provider should set appropriate alarm limits based on the patient's baseline and anticipated physiological parameters.

Step 6: Intraoperative Monitoring Throughout the surgery, the provider should continuously interpret the monitoring data, adjust the anesthesia delivery as needed, and manage any alarms that may occur.

Step 7: Monitor Disconnection At the end of the case, the provider should carefully disconnect the monitors, ensuring patient safety and comfort.

Step 8: Postoperative Check Finally, the provider should perform a postoperative check on each monitor, ensuring it is clean, functional, and ready for the next case.

This step-by-step guide provides detailed instructions for the use of anesthesia monitoring equipment, with defined roles for both the Anesthesia Provider and Anesthesia Technologist. By mastering these processes, the anesthesia team can maximize patient safety and efficacy of care during anesthesia.

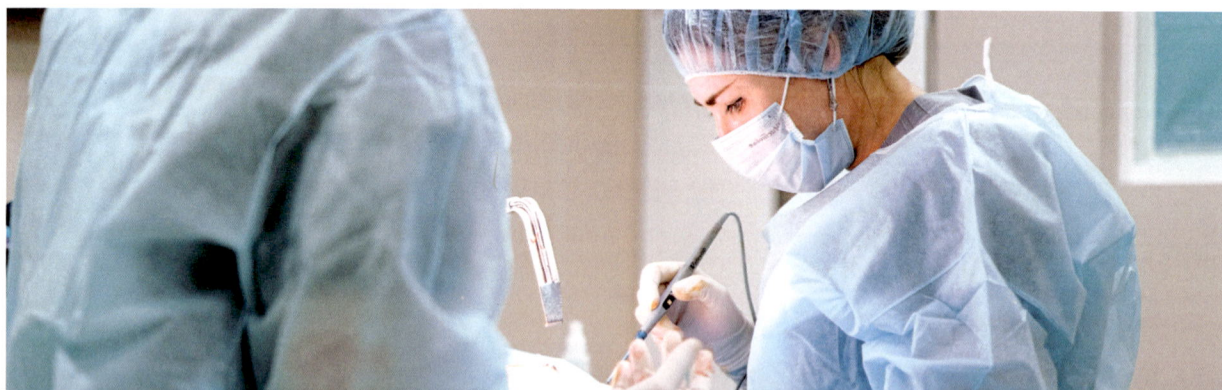

Chapter 6: Airway Management Equipment

In this comprehensive chapter, we will explore the essential topic of airway management equipment. We will provide an overview of various airway management devices, including laryngoscopes, endotracheal tubes, masks, and advanced airway devices. Additionally, we will discuss the proper use, maintenance, and responsibilities of the Anesthesia Provider and Anesthesia Technologist in relation to airway management equipment based on their respective scopes of practice.

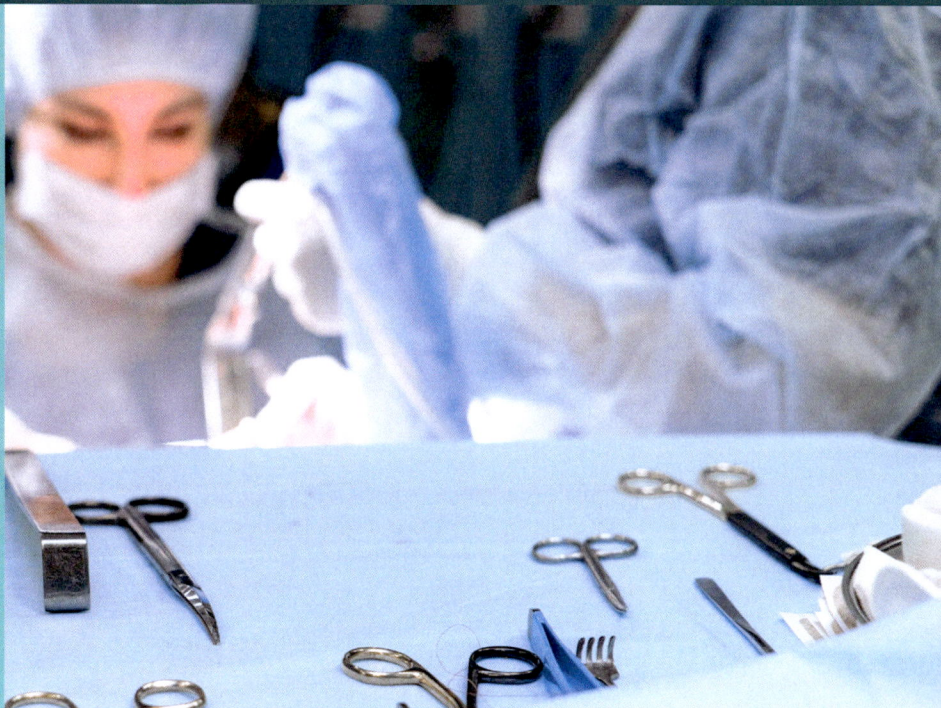

6.1 Overview of Airway Management Devices

Airway management devices are critical tools used to establish and maintain a patent airway during anesthesia procedures. Understanding the different types of airway management devices is crucial for ensuring successful airway management. Let's explore some commonly used devices:

Laryngoscopes: Laryngoscopes are used to visualize the vocal cords and facilitate endotracheal intubation. They consist of a handle and a blade that holds the endotracheal tube. Different types of laryngoscope blades, such as Macintosh and Miller, offer different advantages and are selected based on individual patient anatomy and clinical requirements.

Endotracheal Tubes: Endotracheal tubes are inserted into the patient's trachea to secure the airway and allow for mechanical ventilation. They come in various sizes and materials, such as cuffed or uncuffed, to suit different patient populations and procedures.

Masks: Masks, including facial masks and laryngeal masks, are used to provide positive pressure ventilation and maintain oxygenation during mask ventilation or when a definitive airway cannot be established. They are available in different sizes to ensure an appropriate fit and seal.

Advanced Airway Devices: Advanced airway devices, such as supraglottic airway devices (e.g., laryngeal mask airways, intubating laryngeal mask airways) and video laryngoscopes, offer alternative airway management techniques and assist in challenging airway situations.

DUTIES OF THE ANESTHESIA PROVIDER AND ANESTHESIA TECHNOLOGIST:

The duties and responsibilities of the Anesthesia Provider and Anesthesia Technologist differ based on their scope of practice and institutional policies. Let's examine their roles in relation to airway management equipment:

Anesthesia Provider:

- Selecting the appropriate airway management devices based on the patient's needs, clinical indications, and airway assessment.
- Assessing and managing the patient's airway, including performing direct or video laryngoscopy, endotracheal intubation, or other advanced airway techniques.
- Confirming proper placement and securing of the endotracheal tube.
- Monitoring and maintaining the patient's airway throughout the procedure.
- Collaborating with the Anesthesia Technologist to ensure the availability and proper functioning of airway management equipment.

Anesthesia Technologist:

- Assisting in the setup and preparation of airway management equipment, including laryngoscopes, endotracheal tubes, and masks.
- Ensuring the proper functioning and availability of airway management devices.
- Assisting the Anesthesia Provider during airway interventions, such as passing instruments or assisting with intubation.
- Collaborating with the Anesthesia Provider to ensure the proper cleaning, maintenance, and sterilization of reusable airway management devices.
- Assisting in troubleshooting equipment malfunctions and communicating any concerns or issues to the Anesthesia Provider or appropriate personnel.

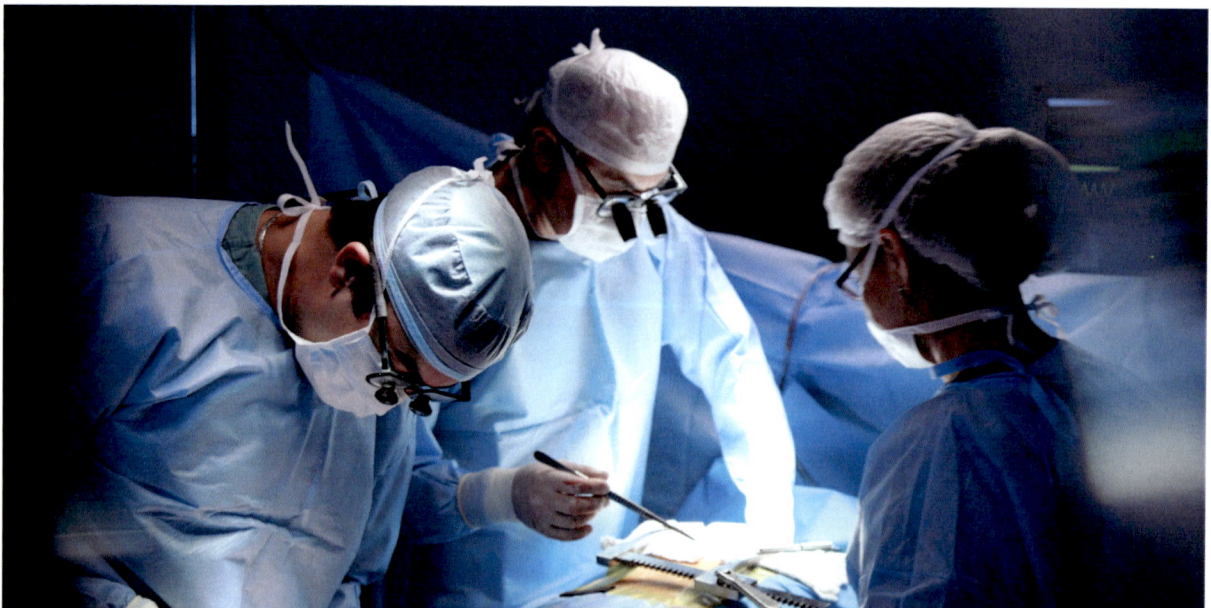

6.2 Proper Use and Maintenance of Laryngoscopes, Endotracheal Tubes, and Masks

Proper use and maintenance of airway management devices are crucial to ensure their safe and effective use. Let's discuss the steps involved in the use and maintenance of laryngoscopes, endotracheal tubes, and masks:

Laryngoscopes:

Ensure the laryngoscope handle is functioning properly, and the batteries are charged or replaced as needed.

Choose the appropriate laryngoscope blade size and type based on patient characteristics and intubation needs.

Perform a pre-use check of the laryngoscope, including inspecting the blade for damage or malfunction.

Lubricate the blade and insert it into the patient's mouth, visualizing the vocal cords to facilitate endotracheal intubation.

Clean and disinfect the laryngoscope after use, following proper infection control protocols.

Endotracheal Tubes:

Select the appropriate size and type of endotracheal tube based on patient characteristics and procedure requirements.

Ensure the integrity of the endotracheal tube, checking for any damage or leaks.

Lubricate the cuff, insert the tube into the patient's trachea, and secure it in place.

Confirm proper tube placement using clinical indicators, such as chest rise, auscultation, and capnography.

Document the size, placement, and any complications related to the endotracheal tube.

Masks:

Select the appropriate mask size and type based on patient characteristics and ventilation needs.

Ensure a proper mask-to-face seal for effective positive pressure ventilation.

Monitor the patient's ventilation and oxygenation during mask ventilation, making adjustments as necessary.

Clean and disinfect reusable masks after use, following proper infection control protocols.

Advanced Airway Devices:

Familiarize yourself with the specific instructions for each advanced airway device, such as laryngeal mask airways or intubating laryngeal mask airways.

Follow the manufacturer's guidelines for insertion, positioning, and securing of the device.

Monitor the patient's ventilation, oxygenation, and airway pressures during the use of advanced airway devices.

Clean and disinfect reusable devices following proper infection control protocols.

DUTIES OF THE ANESTHESIA PROVIDER AND ANESTHESIA TECHNOLOGIST:

Anesthesia Provider:

• Selecting the appropriate airway management devices based on patient factors, clinical indications, and airway assessment.
• Ensuring the safe and effective use of airway management devices, including laryngoscopes, endotracheal tubes, masks, and advanced airway devices.
• Confirming proper placement and securing of the endotracheal tube.
• Monitoring and maintaining the patient's airway throughout the procedure.
• Collaborating with the Anesthesia Technologist to ensure the availability and proper functioning of airway management equipment.

Anesthesia Technologist:

• Assisting in the setup and preparation of airway management equipment, including laryngoscopes, endotracheal tubes, and masks.
• Ensuring the proper functioning and availability of airway management devices.
• Assisting the Anesthesia Provider during airway interventions, such as passing instruments or assisting with intubation.
• Collaborating with the Anesthesia Provider to ensure the proper cleaning, maintenance, and sterilization of reusable airway management devices.
• Assisting in troubleshooting equipment malfunctions and communicating any concerns or issues to the Anesthesia Provider or appropriate personnel.

6.3 Advanced Airway Devices

Advanced airway devices offer additional airway management options, particularly in challenging airway situations. Let's explore some advanced airway devices:

Supraglottic Airway Devices: Supraglottic airway devices, such as laryngeal mask airways (LMAs) and intubating laryngeal mask airways (ILMAs), provide an alternative to traditional endotracheal intubation. They are inserted into the oropharynx, forming a seal over the glottis to facilitate ventilation. These devices are particularly useful in situations where endotracheal intubation may be challenging or contraindicated, such as during short procedures or in patients with difficult airways.

Video Laryngoscopes: Video laryngoscopes provide a visual display of the airway anatomy, aiding in the intubation process. They consist of a camera embedded in the laryngoscope blade, allowing for a clear view of the vocal cords on a monitor. Video laryngoscopes are especially beneficial in patients with limited mouth opening, anatomical abnormalities, or difficult airways.

DUTIES OF THE ANESTHESIA PROVIDER AND ANESTHESIA TECHNOLOGIST:

Anesthesia Provider:

- Selecting the appropriate advanced airway device based on patient factors, airway assessment, and procedural requirements.
- Familiarizing themselves with the proper insertion technique, positioning, and securing of advanced airway devices.
- Monitoring the patient's ventilation, oxygenation, and airway pressures during the use of advanced airway devices.
- Troubleshooting any complications or issues that may arise during the use of advanced airway devices.
- Collaborating with the Anesthesia Technologist to ensure the availability and proper functioning of advanced airway devices.

Anesthesia Technologist:

- Assisting in the setup and preparation of advanced airway devices, ensuring all necessary components are assembled and functioning properly.
- Providing support during the insertion and positioning of advanced airway devices, as guided by the Anesthesia Provider.
- Monitoring the patient's ventilation and oxygenation during the use of advanced airway devices.
- Assisting in troubleshooting any malfunctions or complications related to advanced airway devices.
- Collaborating with the Anesthesia Provider to ensure the proper cleaning, maintenance, and sterilization of reusable advanced airway devices.

By following the proper use, maintenance, and responsibilities outlined in this chapter, anesthesia professionals can ensure safe and effective airway management. It is important to adhere to institutional protocols, manufacturer guidelines, and best practices in order to provide optimal patient care and maintain patient safety throughout the perioperative period.

Chapter 7: Intravenous (IV) and Invasive Line Equipment

In this chapter, we will explore the different types of IV and invasive line equipment used in anesthesia practice. We will discuss the proper setup and operation procedures, as well as maintenance and troubleshooting techniques. Additionally, we will outline the duties of the Anesthesia Provider and the Anesthesia Technologist based on the scope of practice for each type of IV/invasive line.

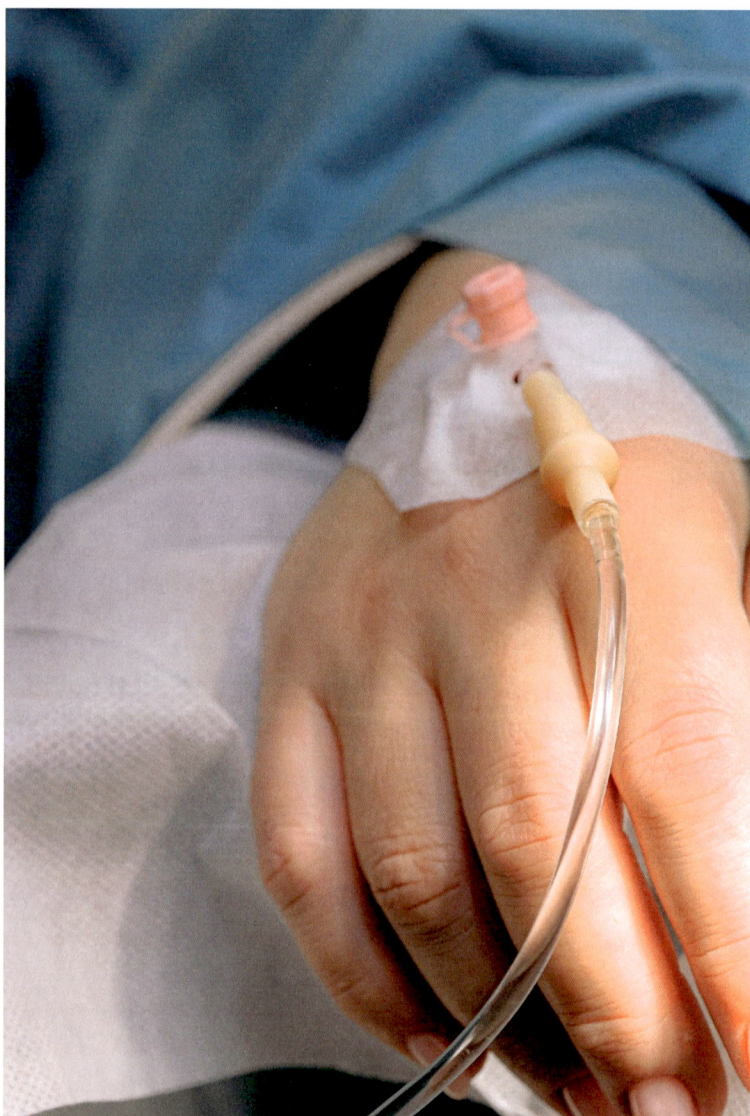

7.1 Different Types of IV and Invasive Line Equipment

There are various types of IV and invasive line equipment used in anesthesia practice. These include:

Peripheral Intravenous (IV) Catheters: These are used for the administration of fluids, medications, and blood products directly into peripheral veins. They are typically inserted into veins in the hand, forearm, or antecubital fossa.

Central Venous Catheters (CVC): These catheters are inserted into large central veins, such as the subclavian, jugular, or femoral veins. They are used for longterm fluid administration, monitoring of central venous pressure, administration of vasoactive medications, and obtaining blood samples.

Arterial Catheters: These catheters are inserted into arteries, usually the radial or femoral artery, for continuous blood pressure monitoring, arterial blood sampling, and access for rapid administration of medications.

Pulmonary Artery Catheters (Swan-Ganz Catheters): These specialized catheters are inserted into the pulmonary artery to measure cardiac output, pulmonary artery pressure, and assess left ventricular function. They are typically used in cardiac and critical care settings.

DUTIES OF THE ANESTHESIA PROVIDER AND ANESTHESIA TECHNOLOGIST:

The duties of the Anesthesia Provider and Anesthesia Technologist may vary based on the scope of practice and local regulations. Here is a breakdown of their responsibilities for each type of IV/invasive line equipment:

Peripheral Intravenous (IV) Catheters:

Anesthesia Provider:

- Selects the appropriate size and gauge of the peripheral IV catheter based on the patient's age, medical condition, and anticipated fluid and medication requirements.
- Inserts the IV catheter using aseptic technique and ensures proper placement.
- Administers fluids, medications, and blood products through the IV catheter.
- Monitors the IV site for signs of infiltration, infection, or other complications.

Anesthesia Technologist:

- Assists with the preparation and setup of the IV equipment, including assembling the IV tubing, priming the tubing with fluids, and connecting the tubing to the IV catheter.
- Maintains aseptic technique during IV setup and assists with securing the IV catheter in place.
- Monitors the IV site for any signs of complications or dislodgement.
- Assists with IV line changes as necessary.

Central Venous Catheters (CVC):

Anesthesia Provider:

- Determines the appropriate site and type of CVC placement based on the patient's condition and medical needs.
- Performs the CVC insertion using sterile technique or guides the placement if performed by an interventional radiologist or surgeon.
- Manages the CVC for fluid administration, medication administration, central venous pressure monitoring, and blood sampling.
- Monitors for any complications related to the CVC, such as infection, thrombosis, or catheter malposition.

Anesthesia Technologist:

- Assists with the preparation and setup of the CVC equipment, including assembling the CVC kit, ensuring proper sterile technique, and connecting the tubing to the CVC.
- Assists with securing the CVC in place and monitoring for proper placement.
- Assists with maintaining the cleanliness and integrity of the CVC dressing and site.
- Assists with CVC removal or line changes as necessary.

Arterial Catheters:

Anesthesia Provider:

- Selects the appropriate arterial site and size of the arterial catheter based on the patient's condition, procedure, and monitoring needs.
- Performs the arterial catheter insertion using sterile technique.
- Calibrates and sets up the arterial pressure monitoring system.
- Monitors the arterial waveform and blood pressure continuously.
- Administers medications through the arterial line as necessary.

Anesthesia Technologist:

- Assists with the preparation and setup of the arterial catheter equipment, including assembling the arterial line kit, ensuring sterile technique, and connecting the tubing to the arterial catheter.
- Assists with securing the arterial catheter in place and monitoring for proper placement.
- Assists with maintaining the cleanliness and integrity of the arterial line dressing and site.
- Assists with arterial line removal or line changes as necessary.

Pulmonary Artery Catheters (Swan-Ganz Catheters):

Anesthesia Provider:

- Determines the need for a pulmonary artery catheter based on the patient's condition and the surgical or critical care requirements.
- Inserts the pulmonary artery catheter using sterile technique or guides the placement if performed by an interventional cardiologist or a trained specialist.
- Monitors the pulmonary artery pressures, cardiac output, and other parameters provided by the catheter.
- Interprets the data obtained and adjusts fluid and medication management accordingly.

Anesthesia Technologist:

- Assists with the preparation and setup of the pulmonary artery catheter equipment, including assembling the catheter kit, ensuring sterile technique, and connecting the monitoring system.
- Assists with positioning the patient and maintaining a sterile field during catheter insertion.
- Assists with maintaining the integrity and proper functioning of the pulmonary artery catheter system.
- Assists with pulmonary artery catheter removal or troubleshooting as necessary.

7.2 Proper Setup and Operation Procedures

Proper setup and operation procedures for IV and invasive line equipment include:

- Ensure a clean and sterile environment when preparing and setting up the equipment.
- Select the appropriate equipment based on the patient's condition, procedure, and monitoring needs.
- Verify the functionality and calibration of the equipment before use.
- Follow aseptic technique during catheter insertion or setup to minimize the risk of infection.
- Secure the catheters in place using appropriate methods and securement devices.
- Connect the tubing to the catheters, ensuring proper connections and priming of the tubing.
- Perform necessary calibrations and zeroing for invasive pressure monitoring systems.
- Monitor the equipment and patient responses closely during operation, making adjustments as necessary.
- Document all relevant information regarding catheter insertion, setup, and operation in the patient's medical record.

7.3 Maintenance and Troubleshooting

Maintenance and troubleshooting of IV and invasive line equipment are vital for ensuring patient safety and optimal performance. Here are some key points:

- Regularly assess the catheter insertion site for signs of complications, such as infection, thrombosis, or dislodgement.

- Maintain the integrity of catheter dressings and securement devices, ensuring they are clean, dry, and intact.
- Follow established protocols for flushing and locking catheters to prevent occlusion or infection.
- Regularly check and replace catheter tubing, pressure monitoring systems, and transducers as per manufacturer guidelines or institutional policies.
- Perform routine inspections of the equipment, including checking for leaks, cracks, or signs of damage.
- Follow a preventive maintenance schedule for equipment, including cleaning, calibration, and functional testing.
- Troubleshoot equipment issues promptly by referring to the manufacturer's guidelines, contacting technical support, or involving biomedical engineering if necessary.
- Document all maintenance and troubleshooting activities in accordance with institutional policies.
- It is essential to recognize the potential consequences if routine maintenance and servicing of IV and invasive line equipment are not performed adequately. Failure to maintain and troubleshoot the equipment can result in various complications, including catheter-related infections, inaccurate pressure monitoring, occlusions, dislodgement, and compromised patient safety.

By understanding the duties of the Anesthesia Provider and Anesthesia Technologist, as well as following proper setup, operation, maintenance, and troubleshooting procedures, anesthesia professionals can ensure the safe and effective use of IV and invasive line equipment. Regular monitoring, documentation, and adherence to protocols and guidelines play a crucial role in maintaining the integrity and functionality of these critical components of anesthesia practice.

7.4 Consequences of Inadequate Maintenance and Servicing

Failure to perform routine maintenance and servicing of IV and invasive line equipment can lead to serious consequences. Here are some potential risks associated with inadequate maintenance:

Infection Risk: Improper maintenance of IV catheters and invasive lines can increase the risk of catheter-related bloodstream infections. Contamination or improper cleaning can introduce bacteria into the bloodstream, leading to local or systemic infections. Infections can result in prolonged hospital stays, increased healthcare costs, and patient discomfort.

Accurate Monitoring Compromised: If invasive pressure monitoring systems, such as arterial or central venous lines, are not properly maintained and calibrated, accurate monitoring of blood pressure, central venous pressure, or other hemodynamic parameters may be compromised. This can lead to inaccurate assessments, delayed interventions, and potential adverse patient outcomes.

Occlusion or Blockage: Failure to flush and maintain patency of IV catheters and invasive lines can result in occlusion or blockage. This can impede the administration of medications, fluids, or blood products, compromising patient care and potentially leading to delays in treatment.

Dislodgement or Malposition: Inadequate securement or monitoring of IV catheters and invasive lines increases the risk of dislodgement or malpositioning. Catheters that are not properly secured or monitored may shift or migrate, potentially causing injury, loss of access, or interruption of therapy.

Equipment Failure: Lack of routine maintenance and servicing can lead to equipment failure. Malfunctioning pressure transducers, faulty tubing, or broken connections can affect the accuracy and reliability of pressure monitoring systems. Equipment failure can result in delayed interventions, inaccurate assessments, and potential patient harm.

Interruption of Therapy: Inadequate maintenance can lead to interruptions in therapy, such as the need for replacement or repair of malfunctioning equipment. This can cause delays in treatment, compromise patient care, and increase healthcare costs.

Increased Risk of Complications: Failure to properly maintain IV and invasive line equipment increases the risk of complications, including thrombosis, embolism, extravasation, or other catheter-related events. These complications can lead to patient discomfort, further interventions, and adverse outcomes.

By understanding the potential consequences of inadequate maintenance and servicing, anesthesia professionals can prioritize the regular maintenance, calibration, and troubleshooting of IV and invasive line equipment. Adhering to institutional policies, manufacturer guidelines, and industry best practices is crucial for ensuring patient safety, optimizing equipment performance, and delivering high-quality anesthesia care.

Note: The specific consequences may vary depending on institutional protocols, equipment used, and local regulations. It is essential to follow the guidelines and recommendations provided by your institution and equipment manufacturers to mitigate risks and ensure patient safety.

Chapter 8: Equipment for Special Anesthesia Applications

This chapter focuses on specialized equipment used in different anesthesia applications, including pediatric anesthesia, obstetric anesthesia, and cardiac anesthesia. Each section will provide a detailed overview of the specific equipment required for these applications, along with the duties breakdown for both the Anesthesia Provider and the Anesthesia Technologist based on their scope of practice.

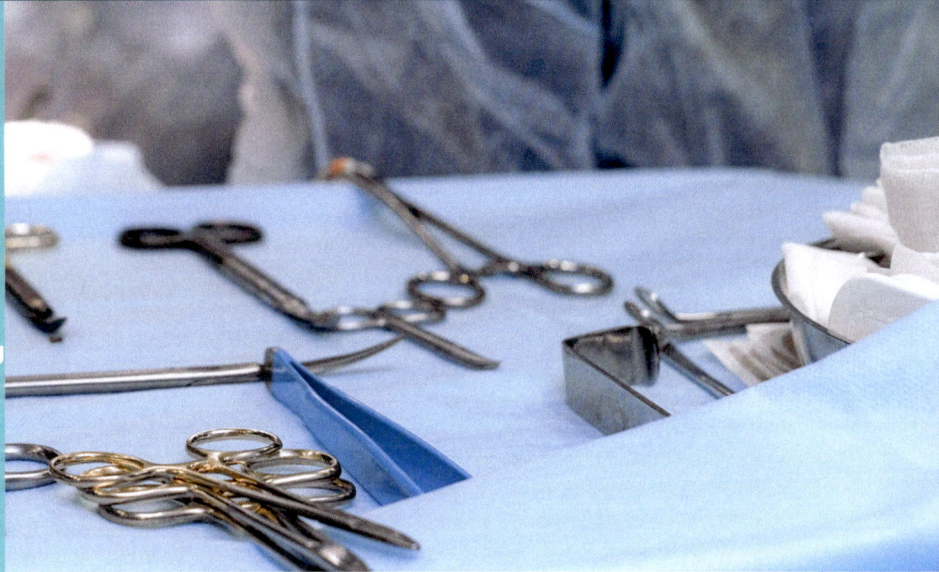

8.1 Equipment for Pediatric Anesthesia

Pediatric anesthesia requires equipment specifically designed to meet the unique needs of infants and children.

DUTIES OF THE ANESTHESIA TECHNOLOGIST:

Step 1: Pediatric-Sized Equipment Preparation: Ensure the availability and proper functioning of pediatric-sized equipment, including masks, endotracheal tubes, laryngoscope blades, breathing circuits, and monitoring devices. Verify that the equipment is appropriately sized for the pediatric patient.

Step 2: Assist with Temperature Regulation: Collaborate with the Anesthesia Provider in maintaining proper temperature regulation for pediatric patients. This may involve using specialized warming devices, such as pediatric-sized warming blankets or radiant warmers.

DUTIES OF THE ANESTHESIA PROVIDER:

Step 3: Pediatric-Specific Airway Management: Select and utilize appropriate airway management techniques and devices for pediatric patients, considering their age, size, and anatomical differences. This may include using smaller-sized laryngoscope blades, endotracheal tubes, or supraglottic airway devices.

Step 4: Monitoring Pediatric Vital Signs: Monitor and interpret vital signs specific to pediatric patients, including heart rate, blood pressure, oxygen saturation, and end-tidal carbon dioxide levels. Utilize pediatric-specific monitoring devices and ensure proper interpretation of age-appropriate reference ranges.

8.2 Equipment for Obstetric Anesthesia

Obstetric anesthesia equipment is tailored to the unique needs of pregnant patients during labor, delivery, and postpartum care.

DUTIES OF THE ANESTHESIA TECHNOLOGIST:

Step 1: Obstetric-Specific Equipment Preparation: Ensure the availability and proper functioning of obstetric-specific equipment, including labor analgesia pumps, epidural trays, intravenous infusion pumps, fetal monitors, and resuscitation equipment for the newborn. Verify that the equipment is in working order and ready for use.

Step 2: Assist with Patient Positioning: Collaborate with the Anesthesia Provider in ensuring proper patient positioning for obstetric procedures. This may involve providing support for the patient's body and limbs, ensuring comfort and stability during the administration of anesthesia.

DUTIES OF THE ANESTHESIA PROVIDER:

Step 3: Epidural and Spinal Anesthesia Administration: Administer epidural or spinal anesthesia for labor analgesia or cesarean section, respectively. Utilize specialized equipment, such as epidural trays, needles, catheters, and infusion pumps, to safely deliver anesthesia and monitor its effects.

Step 4: Fetal Monitoring: Monitor the fetal heart rate and uterine contractions during labor using obstetric-specific fetal monitoring equipment. Interpret fetal heart rate patterns and respond appropriately to any signs of fetal distress.

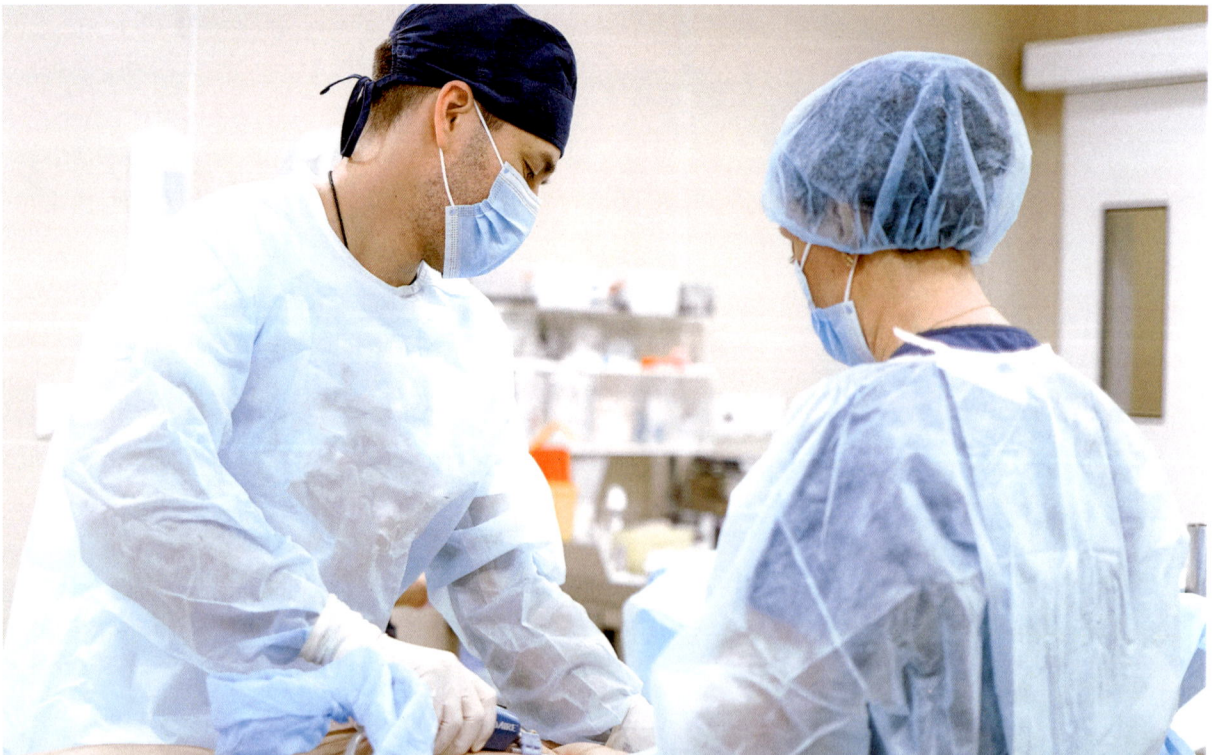

8.3 Equipment for Cardiac Anesthesia

Cardiac anesthesia requires specialized equipment to support the complex procedures performed during cardiac surgery.

DUTIES OF THE ANESTHESIA TECHNOLOGIST:

Step 1: Cardiac-Specific Equipment Preparation: Ensure the availability and proper functioning of cardiac-specific equipment, including transesophageal echocardiography (TEE) probes, invasive monitoring devices (e.g., arterial lines, central venous catheters), cardiopulmonary bypass equipment, and rapid infusion systems for blood products. Verify that all equipment is calibrated and ready for use.

Step 2: Assist with Setup of Cardiopulmonary Bypass: Collaborate with the Anesthesia Provider and the perfusionist in the setup and priming of the cardiopulmonary bypass circuit. Assist with connecting the patient to the bypass machine and ensure proper functioning of all components.

DUTIES OF THE ANESTHESIA PROVIDER:

Step 3: Transesophageal Echocardiography (TEE): Perform TEE during cardiac surgery to provide real-time imaging of the heart and assist in evaluating cardiac function, monitoring valve function, and assessing the adequacy of myocardial protection. Utilize TEE probes and interpret the images obtained.

Step 4: Hemodynamic Management: Monitor and manage hemodynamic parameters during cardiac surgery, including arterial blood pressure, central venous pressure, cardiac output, and mixed venous oxygen saturation. Utilize invasive monitoring devices and interpret the data to optimize patient outcomes.

8.4 Summary

This expanded chapter has provided a comprehensive overview of the specialized equipment used in pediatric anesthesia, obstetric anesthesia, and cardiac anesthesia. By following the step-by-step instructions and understanding the duties of both the Anesthesia Provider and the Anesthesia Technologist, you can ensure the proper preparation, utilization, and monitoring of equipment specific to these applications. Pediatric-sized equipment, temperature regulation, obstetric-specific equipment, patient positioning, cardiac-specific equipment, cardiopulmonary bypass setup, TEE utilization, and hemodynamic management are all critical aspects of providing safe and effective anesthesia care in these specialized settings. By prioritizing these practices, you contribute to optimal patient outcomes and promote excellence in anesthesia delivery.

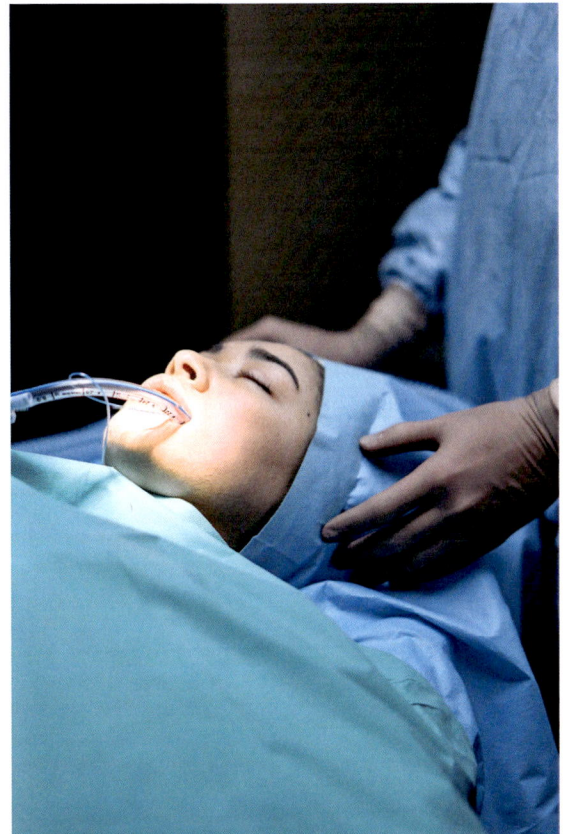

8.5 Equipment for Neurosurgical Anesthesia

Neurosurgical anesthesia requires specialized equipment to support the unique requirements of patients undergoing procedures involving the brain and nervous system.

DUTIES OF THE ANESTHESIA TECHNOLOGIST:

Step 1: Neurosurgical-Specific Equipment Preparation: Ensure the availability and proper functioning of neurosurgical-specific equipment, including neurophysiological monitoring devices, intracranial pressure (ICP) monitoring systems, and brain tissue oxygenation monitors. Verify that the equipment is properly calibrated and ready for use.

Step 2: Assist with Positioning and Head Stabilization: Collaborate with the Anesthesia Provider and the surgical team in positioning the patient and providing adequate head stabilization during neurosurgical procedures. Ensure patient comfort and safety while maintaining optimal access for the surgical team.

DUTIES OF THE ANESTHESIA PROVIDER:

Step 3: Neurophysiological Monitoring: Utilize neurophysiological monitoring devices, such as electroencephalography (EEG), somatosensory evoked potentials (SSEPs), and motor evoked potentials (MEPs), to assess the integrity of the nervous system during surgery. Interpret the data obtained and communicate any significant changes to the surgical team.

Step 4: Intracranial Pressure (ICP) Monitoring: Set up and monitor ICP monitoring systems to assess intracranial dynamics and optimize cerebral perfusion. Utilize specialized ICP monitors and interpret the data obtained to guide management decisions.

8.6 Equipment for Regional Anesthesia

Regional anesthesia techniques require specific equipment to administer local anesthetics and achieve targeted nerve blocks for surgical or pain management purposes.

DUTIES OF THE ANESTHESIA TECHNOLOGIST:

Step 1: Regional Anesthesia Equipment Preparation: Ensure the availability and proper functioning of equipment used for regional anesthesia, including nerve stimulators, ultrasound machines, nerve block trays, and infusion pumps. Verify that the equipment is properly cleaned, calibrated, and ready for use.

Step 2: Assist with Patient Positioning: Collaborate with the Anesthesia Provider and the surgical team in positioning the patient for regional anesthesia procedures. Provide support and assistance to ensure patient comfort and optimal access for the Anesthesia Provider during the nerve block administration.

DUTIES OF THE ANESTHESIA PROVIDER:

Step 3: Nerve Localization and Block Administration: Utilize nerve stimulators or ultrasound guidance to identify the target nerves for regional anesthesia. Administer local anesthetics using specialized needles and catheters to achieve effective nerve blocks. Continuously monitor the patient's response and adjust the technique as needed.

Step 4: Postoperative Pain Management: Utilize infusion pumps and patientcontrolled analgesia (PCA) devices to provide continuous or on-demand delivery of local anesthetics or analgesics for postoperative pain management. Monitor the patient's pain scores and adjust the infusion rates as necessary.

8.7 Summary

This expanded chapter has provided an in-depth understanding of the equipment required for special anesthesia applications, including neurosurgical anesthesia and regional anesthesia. By following the step-by-step instructions and understanding the duties of both the Anesthesia Provider and the Anesthesia Technologist, you can ensure the proper preparation, utilization, and monitoring of equipment specific to these applications. Neurosurgical-specific equipment, neurophysiological monitoring, ICP monitoring, regional anesthesia equipment, nerve localization, and postoperative pain management are crucial aspects of providing safe and effective anesthesia care in these specialized settings. By prioritizing these practices, you contribute to optimal patient outcomes and promote excellence in anesthesia delivery.

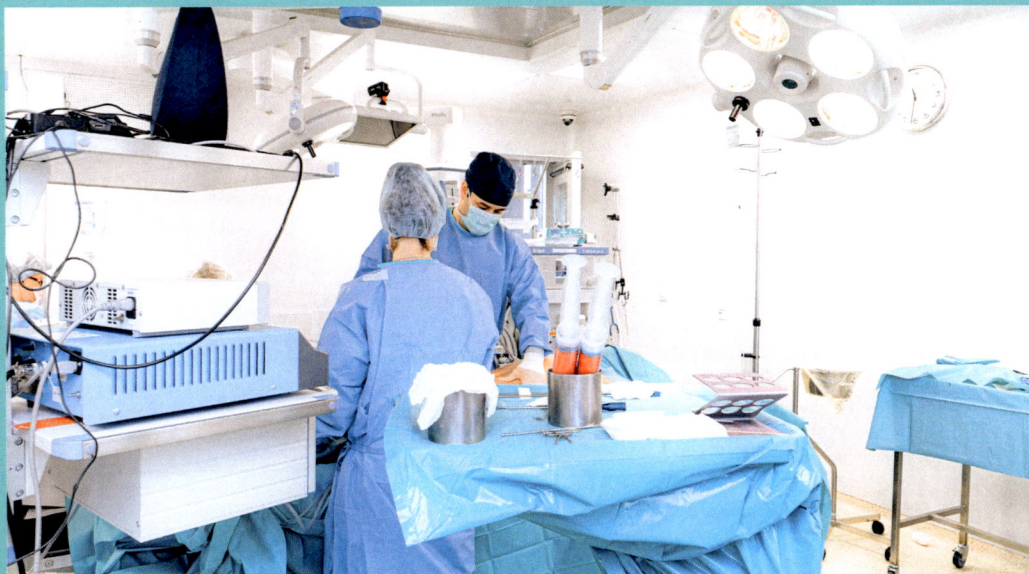

8.8 Equipment for Trauma Anesthesia

Trauma anesthesia requires specialized equipment to manage patients with severe injuries and unstable physiological conditions.

DUTIES OF THE ANESTHESIA TECHNOLOGIST:

Step 1: Trauma-Specific Equipment Preparation: Ensure the availability and proper functioning of trauma-specific equipment, including rapid infusion devices, blood warmers, massive transfusion protocols, and point-of-care testing devices. Verify that the equipment is ready for immediate use and properly calibrated.

Step 2: Assist with Patient Monitoring: Collaborate with the Anesthesia Provider in setting up and maintaining comprehensive patient monitoring during trauma anesthesia. This may involve invasive monitoring of arterial blood pressure, central venous pressure, and arterial blood gas analysis.

DUTIES OF THE ANESTHESIA PROVIDER:

Step 3: Hemorrhage Control and Fluid Resuscitation: Rapidly assess and control bleeding using specialized techniques such as tourniquets, hemostatic agents, or surgical interventions. Administer appropriate fluid resuscitation, blood products, or vasopressor medications to restore hemodynamic stability.

Step 4: Airway Management and Ventilation: Perform advanced airway management techniques, including rapid sequence intubation, in cases of severe trauma. Utilize specialized airway devices, such as video laryngoscopes or bougieassisted intubation, to ensure effective oxygenation and ventilation.

8.9 Equipment for Robotic and Minimally Invasive Surgery

Robotic and minimally invasive surgery requires specific equipment to facilitate precise surgical interventions with minimal patient trauma.

DUTIES OF THE ANESTHESIA TECHNOLOGIST:

Step 1: Robotic and Minimally Invasive-Specific Equipment Preparation: Ensure the availability and proper functioning of equipment specific to robotic and minimally invasive surgery, including patient-side robotic arms, insufflation systems, and specialized monitors. Verify that the equipment is properly calibrated and functioning optimally.

Step 2: Assist with Patient Positioning and Access: Collaborate with the Anesthesia Provider and the surgical team in positioning the patient for robotic or minimally invasive procedures. Ensure patient comfort and stability while allowing the surgical team access to the operative field.

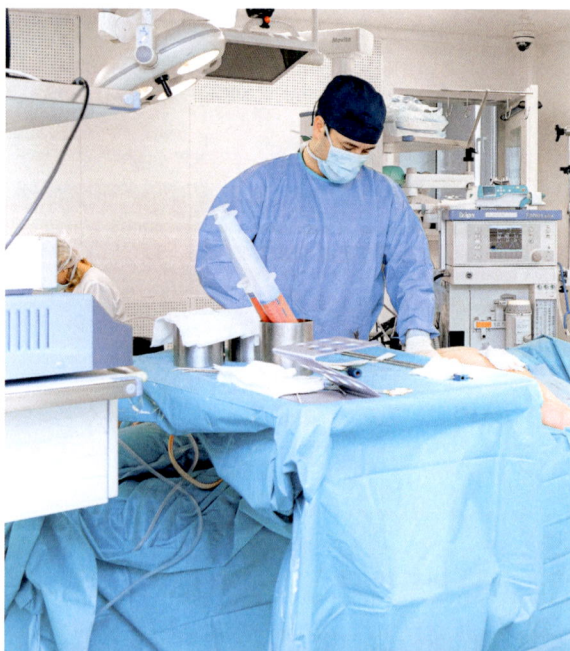

DUTIES OF THE ANESTHESIA PROVIDER:

Step 3: Anesthesia Management for Robotic Surgery: Coordinate anesthesia management with the surgical team, taking into account patient positioning and the specific requirements of the robotic system. Ensure patient safety during pneumoperitoneum creation and optimize ventilation strategies for optimal surgical conditions.

Step 4: Monitoring and Management of Physiological Changes: Continuously monitor the patient's hemodynamic status, end-tidal carbon dioxide levels, and oxygen saturation throughout the robotic or minimally invasive procedure. Respond to any physiological changes promptly to maintain patient stability.

8.10 Summary

This expanded chapter has provided detailed insights into the specialized equipment required for different anesthesia applications, including trauma anesthesia and robotic/minimally invasive surgery. By following the step-by-step instructions and understanding the duties of both the Anesthesia Provider and the Anesthesia Technologist, you can ensure the proper preparation, utilization, and monitoring of equipment specific to these applications. Trauma-specific equipment, hemorrhage control, airway management, robotic/minimally invasive-specific equipment, patient positioning, and anesthesia management for robotic surgery are crucial aspects of providing safe and effective anesthesia care in these specialized settings. By prioritizing these practices, you contribute to optimal patient outcomes and promote excellence in anesthesia delivery.

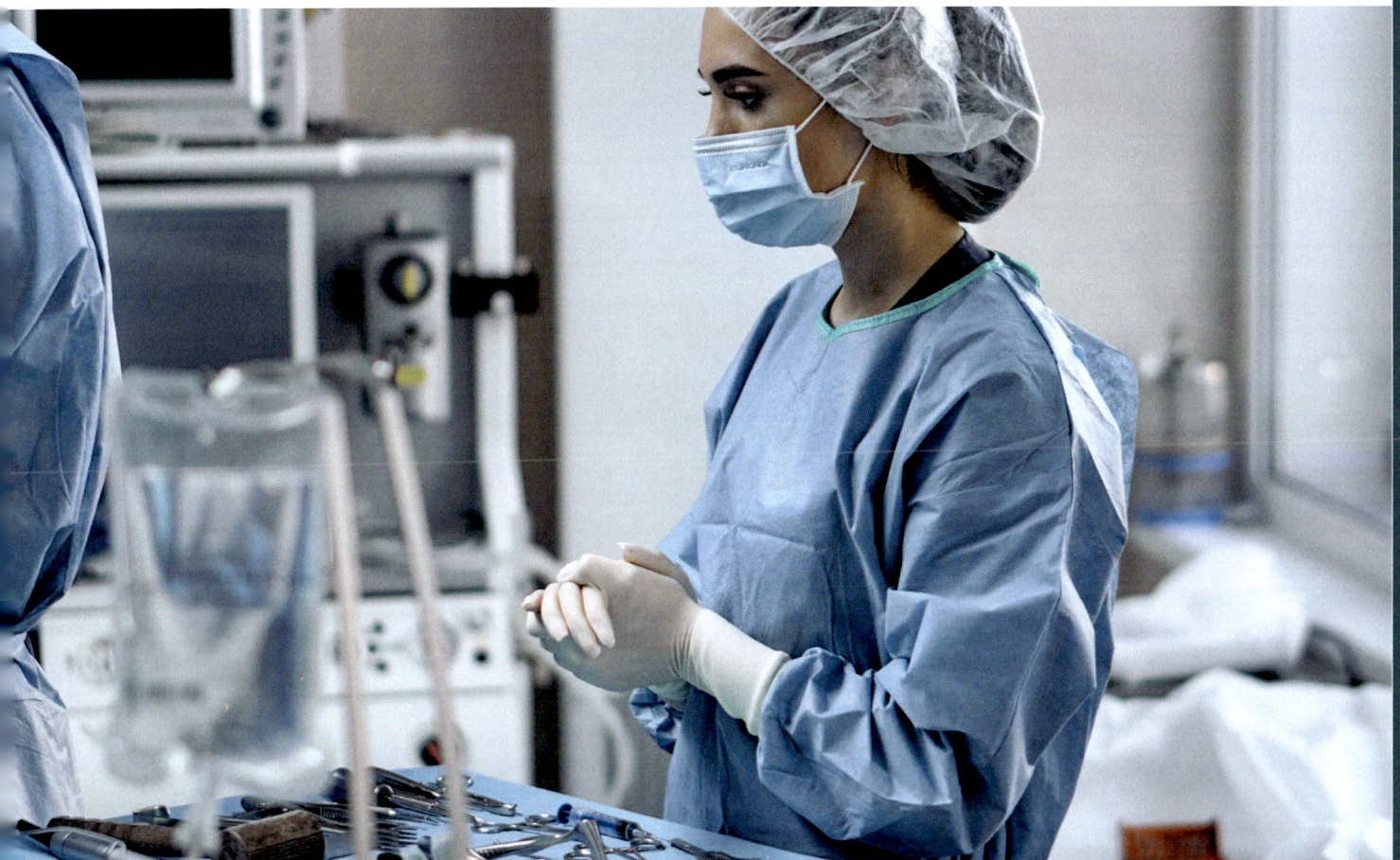

8.11 Equipment for Transplant Anesthesia

Transplant anesthesia requires specialized equipment to support the unique needs of patients undergoing organ transplantation.

DUTIES OF THE ANESTHESIA TECHNOLOGIST:

Step 1: Transplant-Specific Equipment Preparation: Ensure the availability and proper functioning of transplant-specific equipment, including organ preservation solutions, intraoperative monitoring devices, rapid infusion systems, and specialized perfusion devices. Verify that the equipment is properly calibrated and ready for use.

Step 2: Assist with Organ Procurement and Preservation: Collaborate with the Anesthesia Provider and the surgical team in preparing for organ procurement and preservation. This may involve coordinating with organ procurement teams, assisting with the retrieval and preservation of organs, and ensuring proper transport conditions.

DUTIES OF THE ANESTHESIA PROVIDER:

Step 3: Optimize Hemodynamic Stability: Maintain hemodynamic stability during the transplant procedure by utilizing invasive monitoring, adjusting fluid and vasopressor administration, and responding to changes in the patient's physiological status. Continuously assess and optimize organ perfusion to ensure optimal transplant outcomes.

Step 4: Utilize Advanced Monitoring Techniques: Employ advanced monitoring techniques, such as near-infrared spectroscopy (NIRS) or transesophageal echocardiography (TEE), to assess organ perfusion and function during the transplant procedure. Interpret the data obtained and communicate any significant findings to the surgical team.

8.12 Equipment for Remote Anesthesia

Remote anesthesia, also known as tele-anesthesia, utilizes technology to provide anesthesia services in remote or underserved areas.

DUTIES OF THE ANESTHESIA TECHNOLOGIST:

Step 1: Tele-Anesthesia Equipment Preparation: Ensure the availability and proper functioning of tele-anesthesia equipment, including high-quality videoconferencing systems, remote monitoring devices, and secure data transmission platforms. Verify that the equipment is properly set up and tested for connectivity.

Step 2: Assist with Patient Monitoring: Collaborate with the Anesthesia Provider and the remote healthcare team in monitoring the patient's vital signs, anesthesia depth, and other relevant parameters. Provide real-time feedback and assistance to the remote Anesthesia Provider during the procedure.

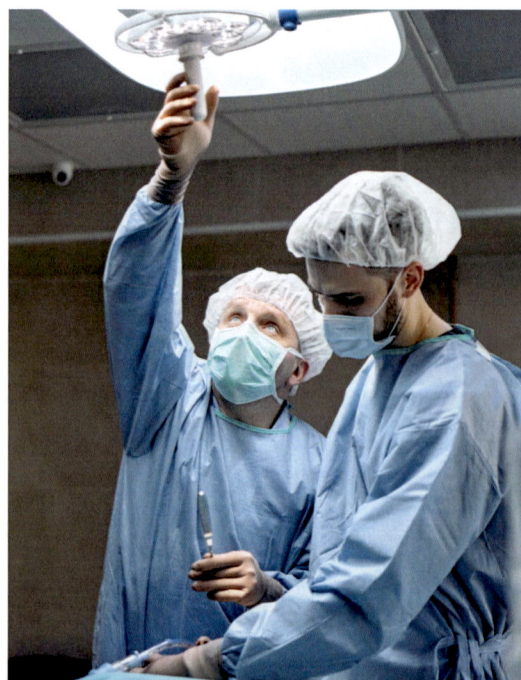

DUTIES OF THE ANESTHESIA PROVIDER:

Step 3: Remote Anesthesia Delivery and Monitoring: Administer anesthesia remotely using videoconferencing and remote monitoring systems. Continuously assess the patient's responses, adjust anesthesia depth and medication administration as needed, and respond to any critical events or emergencies.

Step 4: Ensure Effective Communication: Facilitate clear and effective communication with the remote healthcare team, including the surgical team and nursing staff. Collaborate in decision-making, provide guidance, and ensure seamless coordination of care throughout the remote anesthesia procedure.

8.13 Summary

This expanded chapter has provided detailed information on the specialized equipment required for different anesthesia applications, including transplant anesthesia and remote anesthesia. By following the step-by-step instructions and understanding the duties of both the Anesthesia Provider and the Anesthesia Technologist, you can ensure the proper preparation, utilization, and monitoring of equipment specific to these applications. Transplant-specific equipment, organ procurement and preservation, hemodynamic stability, advanced monitoring techniques, tele-anesthesia equipment, patient monitoring, remote anesthesia delivery, and effective communication are crucial aspects of providing safe and effective anesthesia care in these specialized settings. By prioritizing these practices, you contribute to optimal patient outcomes and promote excellence in anesthesia delivery, even in challenging and remote environments.

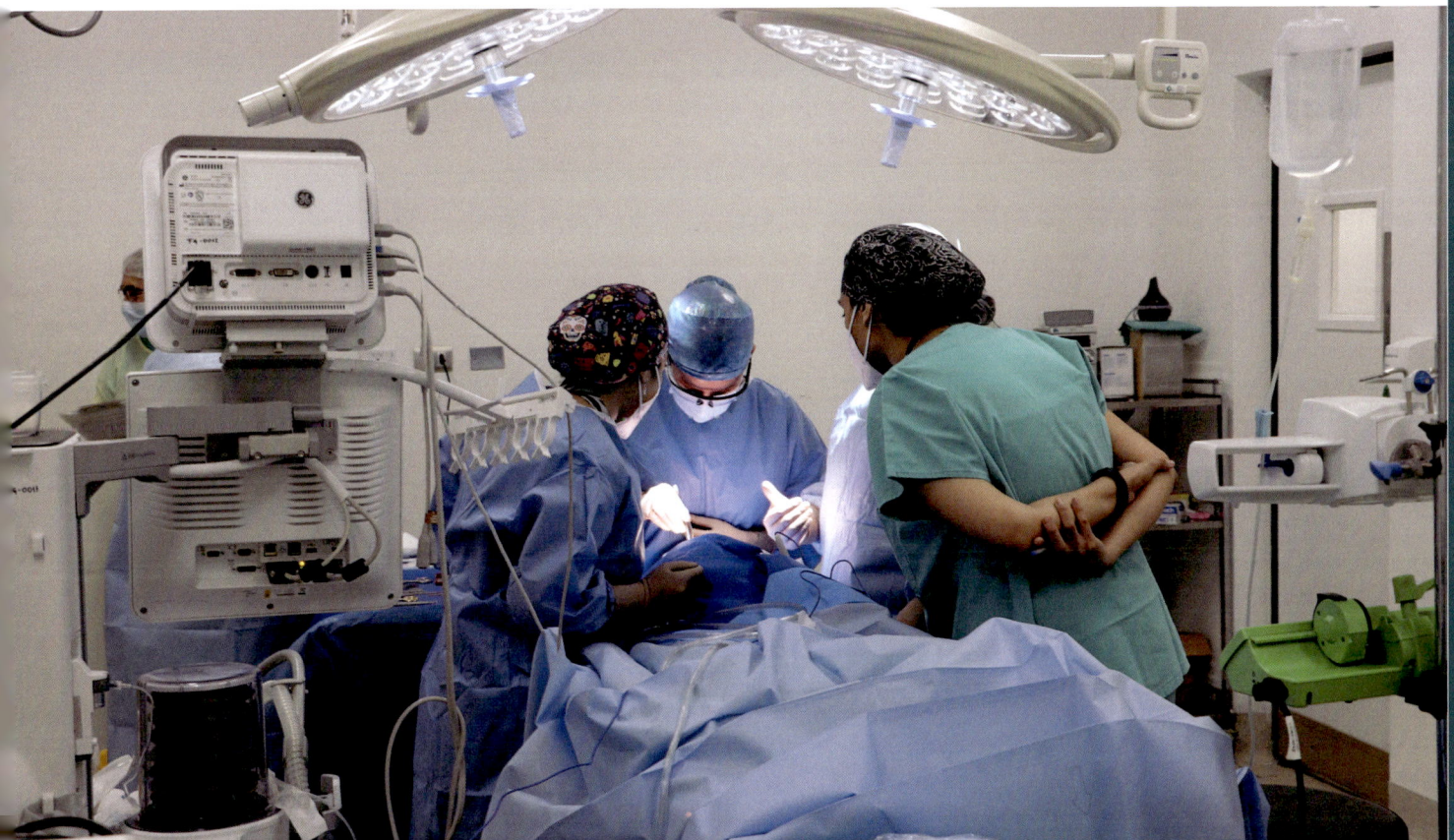

Chapter 9: Comprehensive Breakdown of Troubleshooting Common Anesthesia Equipment Issues

In this expanded guide, we will delve deeper into the common problems that may arise with anesthesia equipment, as well as more comprehensive troubleshooting steps for each problem. We will further outline the duties of the Anesthesia Provider and the Anesthesia Technologist, with added real-world examples to demonstrate the best approach for each problem.

9.1 Anesthesia Machine Problems

9.1.1 High Pressure Alarm

In some scenarios, this could be due to a foreign object obstructing the tubing, or a kink in the circuit. For example, consider a situation where a piece of gauze accidentally made its way into the anesthesia circuit during a surgical procedure.

DUTIES OF THE ANESTHESIA TECHNOLOGIST:

Step 1: Initial Check: If the high-pressure alarm goes off, the Technologist should quickly inspect the circuit for visible blockages or kinks. Check for foreign objects, dislodged parts, or other physical obstructions.

Step 2: Ventilator Check: If there are no visible obstructions and the alarm continues to go off, this could indicate a problem with the ventilator. Check the function of the ventilator, inspecting its connections, controls, and readings.

DUTIES OF THE ANESTHESIA PROVIDER:

Step 3: Patient Assessment: While the Technologist inspects the equipment, the Anesthesia Provider should monitor the patient's vital signs closely, preparing for manual ventilation or alternate ventilation strategies if needed.

9.1.2 Failure of Oxygen Supply

DUTIES OF THE ANESTHESIA TECHNOLOGIST:

Step 1: Oxygen Supply Check: If the oxygen supply suddenly fails during a procedure, check the wall outlet and pipeline pressure gauges. Confirm whether the issue lies with the hospital's central oxygen supply or the specific delivery line.

Step 2: Cylinder Check: If the wall supply fails, the backup oxygen cylinder should kick in. Check the cylinder supply and ensure the cylinder is not empty.

DUTIES OF THE ANESTHESIA PROVIDER:

Step 3: Patient Assessment: Continuously monitor the patient's oxygen saturation level. Be prepared to manually ventilate with an Ambu bag if necessary, and plan for a safe, immediate conclusion of the procedure if the oxygen supply cannot be promptly restored.

9.2 Vaporizer Problems

9.2.1 Over-delivery of Anesthetic Agent

Over-delivery of anesthetic can be a critical issue. It can lead to an overly deep level of anesthesia, hypotension, or respiratory depression.

DUTIES OF THE ANESTHESIA TECHNOLOGIST:

Step 1: Vaporizer Setting Check: The Technologist should first verify the vaporizer settings. Even a small, accidental nudge could result in a dangerous concentration of anesthetic agent being delivered.

Step 2: Seal Check: If the problem persists, inspect the vaporizer for any leakages, particularly around the filler port and vaporizer seals.

DUTIES OF THE ANESTHESIA PROVIDER:

Step 3: Patient Assessment: Monitor the patient's depth of anesthesia and vital signs closely. Be ready to adjust the concentration of anesthetic agent manually or switch to an alternative method if necessary.

9.3 Monitor Problems

9.3.1 Erratic or Inaccurate Readings

Erratic readings can stem from various sources, including electrode or sensor issues, patient factors, or machine malfunction.

DUTIES OF THE ANESTHESIA TECHNOLOGIST:

Step 1: Monitor Calibration: If the readings are erratic, recalibrate the monitor. Monitors should be recalibrated at regular intervals, as per manufacturer guidelines.
Step 2: Lead/Sensor Check: Inspect the leads or sensors for any visible signs of damage or poor contact with the patient.

DUTIES OF THE ANESTHESIA PROVIDER:

Step 3: Patient Assessment: Examine the patient for potential causes such as poor perfusion, movement, or abnormal temperatures that could interfere with accurate readings.

9.4 Ancillary Device Problems

9.4.1 Suction Unit Failure

A suction unit is vital for airway management during anesthetic procedures. Duties of the Anesthesia Technologist:

Step 1: Power Source Check: If the suction unit isn't working, check the power source and connections.
Step 2: Tubing and Container Check: Inspect the suction tubing and collection container for blockages or leaks.

DUTIES OF THE ANESTHESIA PROVIDER:

Step 3: Standby: If troubleshooting is unsuccessful, be prepared to utilize manual suction methods or replace the device as quickly as possible.

This expanded guide gives an in-depth look at troubleshooting common issues with anesthesia equipment. Each issue is paired with real-world examples and a step-by-step guide for both the Anesthesia Provider and Technologist, aiming to ensure the best patient outcomes.

9.5 Issues with Intravenous (IV) Infusion Pumps

9.5.1 Infusion Pump Alarm or Failure

The inability to deliver medication through an infusion pump can have serious implications on the course of an operation.

DUTIES OF THE ANESTHESIA TECHNOLOGIST:

Step 1: Alarm Assessment: Check the display on the infusion pump for any alarm messages. Most infusion pumps provide specific alarm codes which can assist in identifying the problem.
Step 2: Tubing Check: Inspect the IV tubing for kinks or occlusions. Also, verify that the IV catheter site on the patient is patent and not infiltrated.

DUTIES OF THE ANESTHESIA PROVIDER:

Step 3: Alternate Medication Administration: While the Technologist troubleshoots the infusion pump, the Anesthesia Provider should be prepared to manually administer medications if necessary.

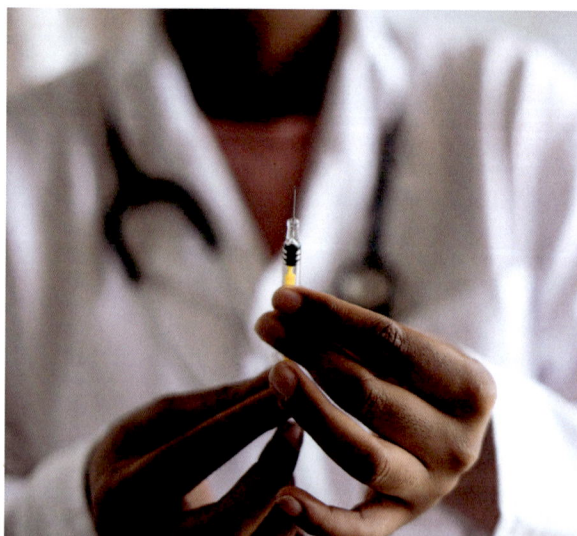

9.6 Advanced Equipment Issues

9.6.1 Problems with Nerve Stimulators

In certain anesthetic procedures, nerve stimulators are employed to facilitate regional anesthesia and monitor depth of neuromuscular blockade.

DUTIES OF THE ANESTHESIA TECHNOLOGIST:

Step 1: Battery and Connection Check: Ensure that the battery is not dead and all connections are secure.

Step 2: Electrode Check: Check the integrity and placement of the electrodes on the patient. The stimulator might fail to work if the electrodes are not correctlyplaced.

DUTIES OF THE ANESTHESIA PROVIDER:

Step 3: Clinical Assessment: While the Technologist checks the equipment, the Anesthesia Provider should reassess the level of blockade using clinical indicators and be prepared to modify the anesthesia plan accordingly.

9.7 Anesthesia Information Management Systems (AIMS) Issues

9.7.1 Software Failure or Data Loss

AIMS are computer systems that collect, store, and display patient data. Any failure in these systems can disrupt workflow and patient monitoring.

DUTIES OF THE ANESTHESIA TECHNOLOGIST:

Step 1: Initial Software Troubleshooting: Check for error messages and perform a basic software restart if necessary.

Step 2: IT Support: If problems persist, involve the IT department promptly. Backup the data, if possible, to avoid loss.

DUTIES OF THE ANESTHESIA PROVIDER:

Step 3: Manual Charting and Patient Monitoring: If the AIMS is down, the Anesthesia Provider will need to revert to manual patient charting and possibly adjust patient monitoring strategies.

By breaking down common equipment issues and troubleshooting steps for both the Anesthesia Provider and Anesthesia Technologist, this guide provides a comprehensive look at the various problems that may occur in the operating room. It is crucial to remember that in addition to these troubleshooting steps, immediate consultation with the bioengineering department or equipment manufacturer may be necessary for more complex issues or when initial troubleshooting fails.

9.8 Airway Management Equipment Issues

9.8.1 Laryngoscope Failure

Failure of the laryngoscope, used for endotracheal intubation, can disrupt an anesthetic procedure and complicate airway management.

DUTIES OF THE ANESTHESIA TECHNOLOGIST:

Step 1: Battery and Bulb Check: If the laryngoscope isn't working, the first step is to check the battery and bulb.
Step 2: Contact Check: Ensure that the bulb is screwed in tightly, and the contact between the bulb and battery is not compromised.

DUTIES OF THE ANESTHESIA PROVIDER:

Step 3: Alternate Laryngoscope or Intubation Device: If the laryngoscope fails, the Provider should immediately opt for an alternative laryngoscope or other intubation devices.

9.9 Anesthesia Circuit Problems

9.9.1 Leak in the Anesthesia Circuit

Leaks can cause loss of anesthetic gases, compromise ventilation, and risk environmental pollution with volatile anesthetics.

DUTIES OF THE ANESTHESIA TECHNOLOGIST:

Step 1: Visual and Auditory Check: A preliminary check involves visually inspecting the circuit and listening for the distinctive sound of a gas leak.
Step 2: Pressure Check: Apply pressure to the system using the ventilation bag while occluding the patient end of the circuit. Observe the pressure gauge to see if it holds steady, which will help locate a leak.

DUTIES OF THE ANESTHESIA PROVIDER:

Step 3: Manual Ventilation and Patient Monitoring: While the Technologist is troubleshooting, the Anesthesia Provider should take over manual ventilation and closely monitor the patient's vitals.

9.10 Waste Anesthetic Gas Disposal (WAGD) System Issues

9.10.1 Insufficient or Failed Scavenging of Anesthetic Gases

The scavenging system reduces occupational exposure to waste anesthetic gases. Failure can risk overexposure to these gases.

DUTIES OF THE ANESTHESIA TECHNOLOGIST:

Step 1: Scavenger Interface Check: Verify that the scavenger interface is connected properly and that the relief ports are not obstructed.

Step 2: Gas Collection Assembly Check: Examine the tubing, gas collection bag, and connections for any leaks.

DUTIES OF THE ANESTHESIA PROVIDER:

Step 3: Minimize Anesthetic Gas Release: Limit the release of anesthetic gases as much as possible and alert the operating room team of potential overexposure until the system is fixed.

The chapter continues to address other potential equipment issues and outlines the step-by-step process to tackle each one. With this guide, both the Anesthesia Provider and Anesthesia Technologist can work effectively as a team to ensure the smooth running of the anesthesia delivery and monitoring system.

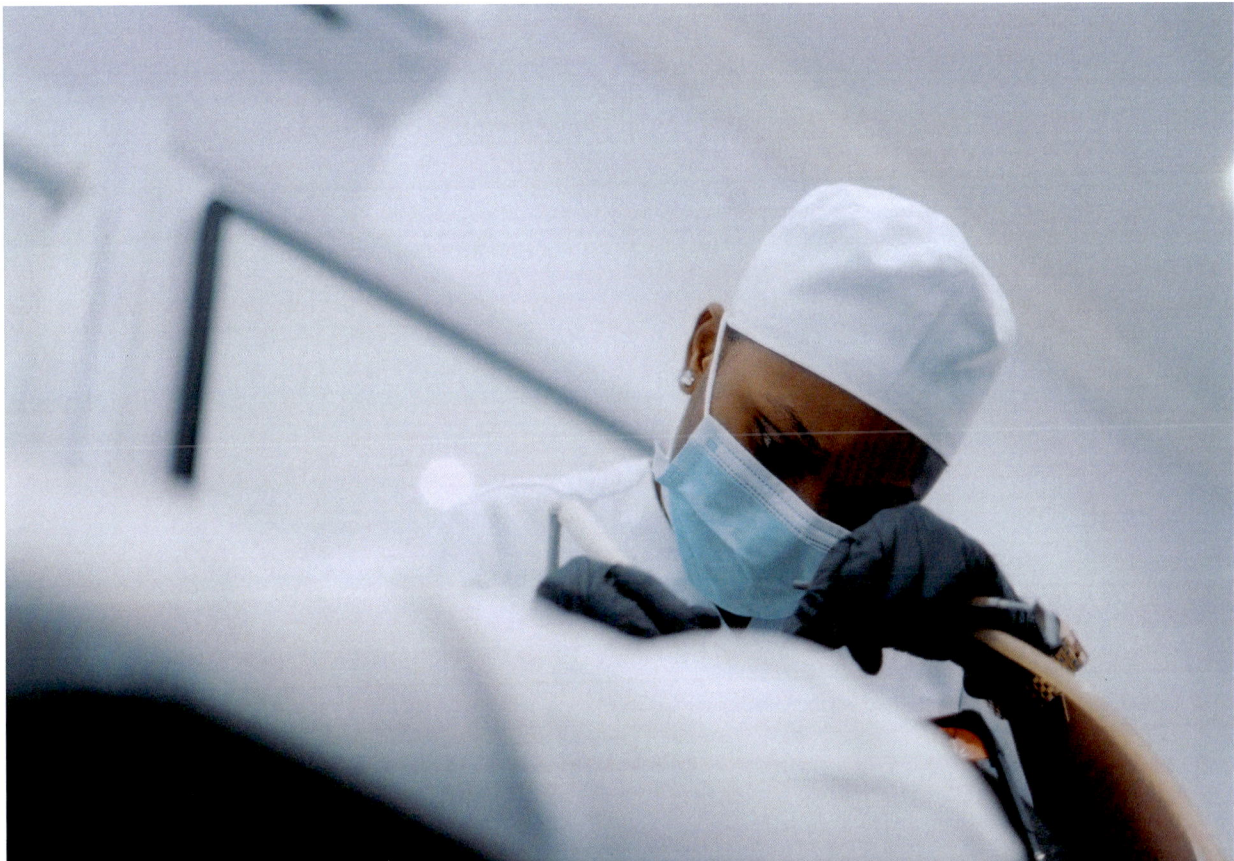

Chapter 10: Ensuring Patient Safety and Emergency Preparedness in Anesthesia

In this chapter, we will provide step-by-step instructions on how to ensure patient safety and be prepared for emergencies during anesthesia procedures. The duties and responsibilities of both the Anesthesia Provider and the Anesthesia Technologist will be outlined to ensure a comprehensive approach to patient care.

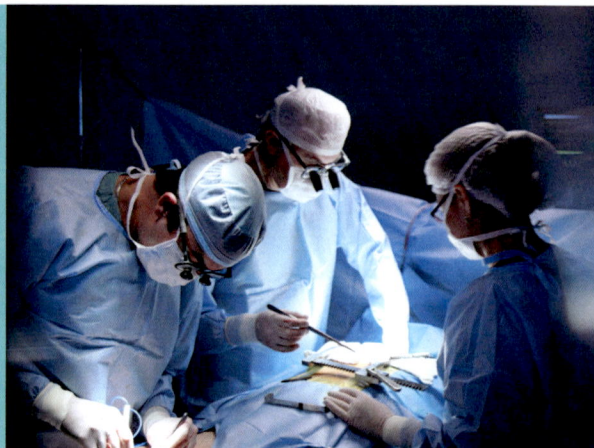

10.1 Preoperative Patient Assessment

DUTIES OF THE ANESTHESIA PROVIDER:

Step 1: Review Patient's Medical History: Thoroughly review the patient's medical history, including allergies, previous anesthetic experiences, and any comorbidities that may affect anesthesia.
Step 2: Perform a Physical Examination: Conduct a comprehensive physical examination to assess the patient's overall health status, airway anatomy, and cardiovascular function.

DUTIES OF THE ANESTHESIA TECHNOLOGIST:

Step 3: Assist with Data Collection: Assist the Anesthesia Provider in collecting and documenting relevant patient data, such as vital signs, laboratory results, and diagnostic imaging.

10.2 Ensuring a Safe Anesthetic Environment

DUTIES OF THE ANESTHESIA TECHNOLOGIST:

Step 1: Prepare the Anesthetic Workspace: Set up the anesthesia machine, ensuring all necessary equipment, supplies, and medications are readily accessible.
Step 2: Perform Equipment Checks: Conduct routine checks of the anesthesia machine, monitors, and other equipment to ensure proper functioning and calibration.

DUTIES OF THE ANESTHESIA PROVIDER:

Step 3: Verify Medications and Equipment: Cross-check medication labels and verify proper functioning of equipment, including anesthesia circuits, endotracheal tubes, and airway devices.

10.3 Anesthetic Induction and Maintenance

DUTIES OF THE ANESTHESIA PROVIDER:

Step 1: Administer Induction Agents: Safely administer induction agents, such as intravenous anesthetics or inhalational agents, while closely monitoring the patient's vital signs and level of consciousness.

Step 2: Establish Airway Management: Secure the patient's airway through intubation or other appropriate airway management techniques based on the patient's specific needs.

DUTIES OF THE ANESTHESIA TECHNOLOGIST:

Step 3: Assist with Airway Management: Provide assistance during airway management procedures, ensuring proper positioning, suctioning, and documentation of the procedure.

10.4 Intraoperative Monitoring and Support

DUTIES OF THE ANESTHESIA PROVIDER:

Step 1: Monitor Vital Signs: Continuously monitor the patient's vital signs, including blood pressure, heart rate, oxygen saturation, and end-tidal carbon dioxide levels.

Step 2: Adjust Anesthetic Agents: Titrate anesthetic agents to maintain an appropriate depth of anesthesia, analgesia, and hemodynamic stability throughout the procedure.

DUTIES OF THE ANESTHESIA TECHNOLOGIST:

Step 3: Assist with Monitoring and Documentation: Assist in monitoring and documenting vital signs, input/output measurements, and any other pertinent data during the procedure.

10.5 Emergencies and Crisis Management

DUTIES OF THE ANESTHESIA PROVIDER:

Step 1: Recognize and Assess Emergencies: Quickly recognize signs of emergencies such as anaphylaxis, malignant hyperthermia, or cardiovascular collapse. Assess the severity of the situation and initiate appropriate interventions.

Step 2: Coordinate the Emergency Response: Direct the team's response to the emergency, ensuring proper communication, assigning tasks, and requesting necessary assistance from other healthcare professionals.

DUTIES OF THE ANESTHESIA TECHNOLOGIST:

Step 3: Assist with Emergency Procedures: Provide immediate assistance during emergency procedures, including cardiopulmonary resuscitation (CPR), defibrillation, and administration of emergency medications as directed by the Anesthesia Provider.

10.6 Postoperative Patient Care

DUTIES OF THE ANESTHESIA TECHNOLOGIST:

Step 1: Transfer to Post-Anesthesia Care Unit (PACU): Assist with the safe transfer of the patient to the PACU, ensuring proper monitoring and continuity of care during the handover process.

DUTIES OF THE ANESTHESIA PROVIDER:

Step 2: Post-Anesthetic Evaluation: Conduct a thorough post-anesthetic evaluation, assessing the patient's recovery, vital signs, pain management needs, and readiness for discharge from the PACU.

10.7 Summary

This chapter has provided a detailed guide on ensuring patient safety and emergency preparedness in anesthesia. By understanding and following the stepby-step instructions outlined for the Anesthesia Provider and Anesthesia Technologist, you can effectively contribute to providing high-quality care, minimizing risks, and responding appropriately to emergencies during anesthesia procedures.

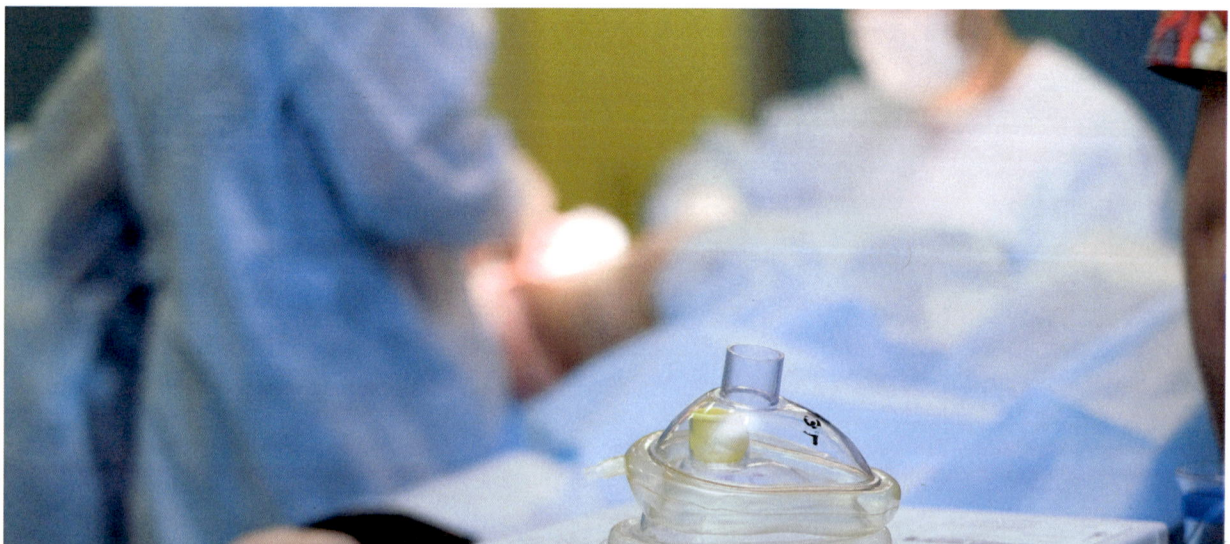

10.8 Documentation and Communication

DUTIES OF THE ANESTHESIA TECHNOLOGIST:

Step 1: Record Keeping: Maintain accurate and detailed documentation of all procedures, medications administered, monitoring parameters, and any significant events or interventions during the anesthesia procedure.

DUTIES OF THE ANESTHESIA PROVIDER:

Step 2: Handover and Communication: Effectively communicate with the postanesthesia care unit (PACU) staff, providing a comprehensive handover report that includes important patient information, intraoperative events, and any ongoing concerns or considerations.

10.9 Continuous Professional Development and Quality Improvement

DUTIES OF THE ANESTHESIA TECHNOLOGIST:

Step 1: Stay Updated: Engage in continuous professional development by staying updated on current best practices, guidelines, and technological advancements in anesthesia care.

DUTIES OF THE ANESTHESIA PROVIDER:

Step 2: Participate in Quality Improvement Initiatives: Actively participate in quality improvement initiatives, such as morbidity and mortality conferences, root cause analysis, and implementation of evidence-based practices to enhance patient safety and outcomes.

10.10 Conclusion

By following the step-by-step instructions provided for the Anesthesia Provider and Anesthesia Technologist in this chapter, you can ensure patient safety and be prepared to handle emergencies during anesthesia procedures. It is essential to collaborate as a team, communicate effectively, and maintain a commitment to continuous professional development and quality improvement.

By adhering to these practices, you can contribute to providing optimal anesthesia care and fostering a culture of patient safety.

10.11 Infection Control and Sterile Techniques

DUTIES OF THE ANESTHESIA TECHNOLOGIST:

Step 1: Hand Hygiene and Personal Protective Equipment (PPE): Adhere to proper hand hygiene practices and wear appropriate PPE, including gloves, masks, and gowns, to prevent the spread of infection.

Step 2: Equipment Sterilization and Disinfection: Follow established protocols for sterilizing and disinfecting anesthesia equipment, ensuring that all surfaces and reusable items are properly cleaned between patient uses.

DUTIES OF THE ANESTHESIA PROVIDER:

Step 3: Aseptic Technique: Utilize aseptic technique when performing invasive procedures, such as central line placement or regional anesthesia, to minimize the risk of introducing pathogens into the patient's body.

10.12 Anesthesia Machine and Equipment Safety Checks

DUTIES OF THE ANESTHESIA TECHNOLOGIST:

Step 1: Pre-Procedure Checks: Conduct thorough safety checks of the anesthesia machine and related equipment before each procedure. This includes inspecting the machine for visible damage, ensuring proper functioning of alarms, and confirming adequate supply of oxygen and other gases.

Step 2: Equipment Functionality Tests: Perform routine functionality tests, such as verifying proper functioning of flowmeters, vaporizers, and ventilators, to ensure that all components are in working order.

DUTIES OF THE ANESTHESIA PROVIDER:

Step 3: Critical Event Preparedness: Familiarize yourself with emergency procedures and protocols specific to the anesthesia machine and equipment, such as power failure or machine malfunction. Ensure that backup systems and supplies are readily available.

10.13 Maintaining a Safe Medication Administration Process

DUTIES OF THE ANESTHESIA TECHNOLOGIST:

Step 1: Medication Preparation: Assist in medication preparation, ensuring accuracy in drug selection, calculation, and labeling. Adhere to proper aseptic techniques during medication handling.

Step 2: Double-Check Process: Engage in the double-check process, where two healthcare professionals verify the medication, concentration, and dosage before administration.

DUTIES OF THE ANESTHESIA PROVIDER:

Step 3: Safe Medication Administration: Administer medications safely, following the five rights of medication administration: right patient, right drug, right dose, right route, and right time.

10.14 Patient Advocacy and Communication

DUTIES OF THE ANESTHESIA TECHNOLOGIST:

Step 1: Patient Education: Provide patients with clear and concise information regarding the anesthesia process, potential risks, and what to expect during their procedure.

Step 2: Support Patient Comfort and Safety: Assist in positioning the patient comfortably and ensuring that safety measures, such as securing limbs and protecting pressure points, are implemented.

DUTIES OF THE ANESTHESIA PROVIDER:

Step 3: Informed Consent: Engage in informed consent discussions with the patient, explaining the risks, benefits, and alternatives of anesthesia, and addressing any questions or concerns they may have.

10.15 Summary

This chapter has provided a detailed guide on ensuring patient safety and emergency preparedness in anesthesia, with specific duties outlined for both the Anesthesia Provider and Anesthesia Technologist. By following these step-by-step instructions, you can contribute to a safe and efficient anesthesia practice, promoting positive patient outcomes and effective communication within the healthcare team. By prioritizing infection control, equipment safety, medication administration, patient advocacy, and continuous improvement, you can provide exceptional care and ensure patient safety throughout the anesthesia process.

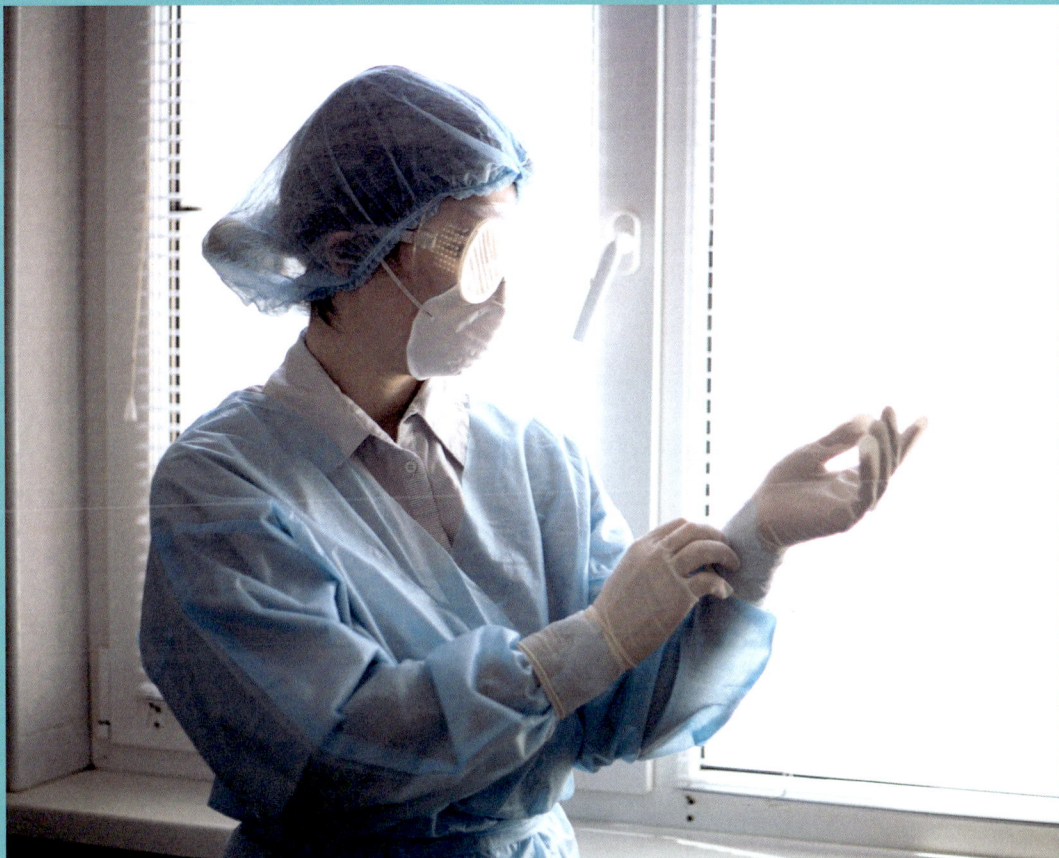

Chapter 11: Future Trends in Anesthesia Equipment

In this chapter, we will explore the exciting realm of future trends in anesthesia equipment. As technology continues to advance, anesthesia professionals must stay informed about the latest developments and prepare for the changes ahead. We will delve into technological advancements, the impact of artificial intelligence, and strategies for adapting to future changes in anesthesia practice.

Let's dive in:

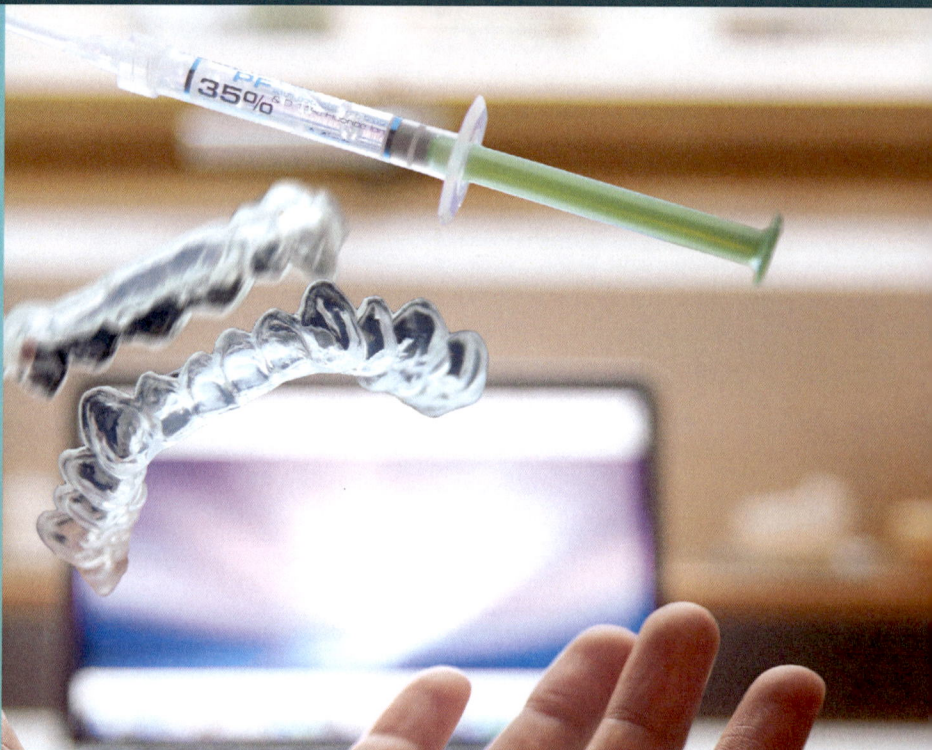

11.1 Technological Advancements in Anesthesia Equipment

Technology plays a pivotal role in shaping the field of anesthesia, improving patient outcomes, and enhancing workflow efficiency. Let's examine some of the significant technological advancements in anesthesia equipment:

Monitoring and Data Integration: Future anesthesia equipment will feature advanced monitoring capabilities that integrate various parameters into a comprehensive data set. This includes real-time monitoring of vital signs, depth of anesthesia, hemodynamic parameters, and neurological status. Anesthesia providers will be able to access this integrated data for enhanced decision-making and individualized patient care.

Smart Infusion Systems: Infusion pumps will become smarter, incorporating features such as closed-loop feedback systems and drug libraries to ensure precise medication administration. These systems will integrate with patient monitoring, allowing for automated adjustments based on individual patient needs and responses.

Wireless Connectivity: Anesthesia equipment will increasingly utilize wireless connectivity, allowing seamless integration with electronic health records (EHRs) and other hospital systems. This connectivity facilitates real-time data sharing, remote monitoring, and improved communication among healthcare providers.

Enhanced Imaging and Visualization: Advancements in imaging technologies will provide anesthesia providers with improved visualization during procedures. This includes high-resolution displays, three-dimensional imaging, and augmented reality/virtual reality applications for preoperative planning and intraoperative guidance.

DUTIES OF THE ANESTHESIA PROVIDER AND ANESTHESIA TECHNOLOGIST:

Anesthesia Provider:

- Staying informed about technological advancements in anesthesia equipment. Embracing and adapting to new equipment and technologies in clinical practice.
- Participating in training programs to learn how to effectively use advanced equipment.
- Collaborating with biomedical engineering or IT departments to ensure seamless integration of new technologies into practice.
- Providing feedback on equipment usability, functionality, and performance to manufacturers and developers.

Anesthesia Technologist:

- Staying updated on technological advancements and changes in anesthesia equipment.
- Assisting the Anesthesia Provider in the setup, operation, and troubleshooting of advanced equipment.
- Participating in training programs to enhance technical skills and understanding of new technologies.
- Collaborating with the Anesthesia Provider and biomedical engineering to ensure proper maintenance and utilization of advanced equipment.
- Providing input and feedback on equipment performance and usability.

11.2 The Impact of Artificial Intelligence on Anesthesia Equipment

Artificial intelligence (AI) has the potential to revolutionize anesthesia practice by augmenting decision-making, improving patient safety, and enhancing workflow efficiency. Let's explore the impact of AI on anesthesia equipment:

Anesthesia Decision Support Systems: AI algorithms can analyze patient data, monitor trends, and provide real-time recommendations to aid anesthesia providers in decision-making. This includes optimizing drug dosages, predicting patient responses, and alerting to potential complications.

Machine Learning in Anesthesia Monitoring: Machine learning algorithms can analyze large datasets and learn patterns to provide predictive analytics in anesthesia monitoring. This can assist in identifying subtle changes in patient physiology, alerting to potential adverse events, and optimizing anesthesia delivery.

Automation and Robotics: AI-powered automation and robotics can streamline routine tasks, such as medication preparation, device setup, and data entry, freeing up anesthesia providers to focus on patient care. Robotic assistance can also enhance precision and dexterity during complex procedures. Duties of the Anesthesia Provider and Anesthesia Technologist:

Anesthesia Provider:

- Staying informed about the advancements and applications of AI in anesthesia practice.
- Collaborating with AI developers and researchers to provide feedback on AIdriven decision support systems.
- Understanding the limitations and potential biases of AI algorithms to make informed clinical decisions.
- Participating in training programs to effectively utilize AI-driven technologies.
- Ensuring the ethical use of AI in anesthesia practice and maintaining patientcentered care.

Anesthesia Technologist:

- Staying updated on the integration of AI technologies in anesthesia equipment.
- Assisting the Anesthesia Provider in the setup, calibration, and operation of AIdriven equipment.

- Collaborating with biomedical engineering or IT departments to ensure proper integration of AI technologies.
- Participating in training programs to enhance technical skills and understanding of AI-driven equipment.
- Providing input and feedback on the usability and functionality of AI technologies.

11.3 Preparing for Future Changes in Anesthesia Practice

As anesthesia practice evolves, it is crucial for anesthesia professionals to proactively prepare for future changes. Here are some strategies to adapt to the evolving landscape:

Continuing Education and Professional Development: Engage in ongoing education and professional development to stay updated on advancements and changes in anesthesia practice. Attend conferences, workshops, and courses that focus on emerging technologies and future trends.

Collaboration and Interdisciplinary Communication: Foster collaboration with other healthcare providers and departments to understand evolving patient needs and incorporate new technologies effectively. Participate in interdisciplinary forums and committees to shape the future of anesthesia practice.

Embracing Change and Adopting New Technologies: Embrace a growth mindset and be open to adopting new technologies and practices. Actively seek opportunities to learn and gain proficiency in using emerging anesthesia equipment and technologies.

Participating in Research and Innovation: Contribute to research and innovation in anesthesia practice by participating in clinical trials, quality improvement projects, and technological advancements. Actively seek opportunities to contribute to the development and evaluation of new equipment and techniques.

Advocacy and Leadership: Advocate for the integration of new technologies and best practices in anesthesia practice. Take on leadership roles within professional organizations or institutional committees to drive change and promote innovation.

By actively preparing for future changes, anesthesia professionals can ensure that they remain at the forefront of advancements, deliver high-quality patient care, and contribute to the ongoing improvement of anesthesia practice.

Remember, as technology continues to evolve, it is important to maintain a balance between embracing innovation andadhering to patient safety principles and ethical considerations. Stay informed, adapt to new technologies, and continuously strive for excellence in providing anesthesia care. The future of anesthesia equipment holds exciting possibilities, and by staying proactive and prepared, anesthesia professionals can shape the future of the field and continue delivering optimal care to their patients.

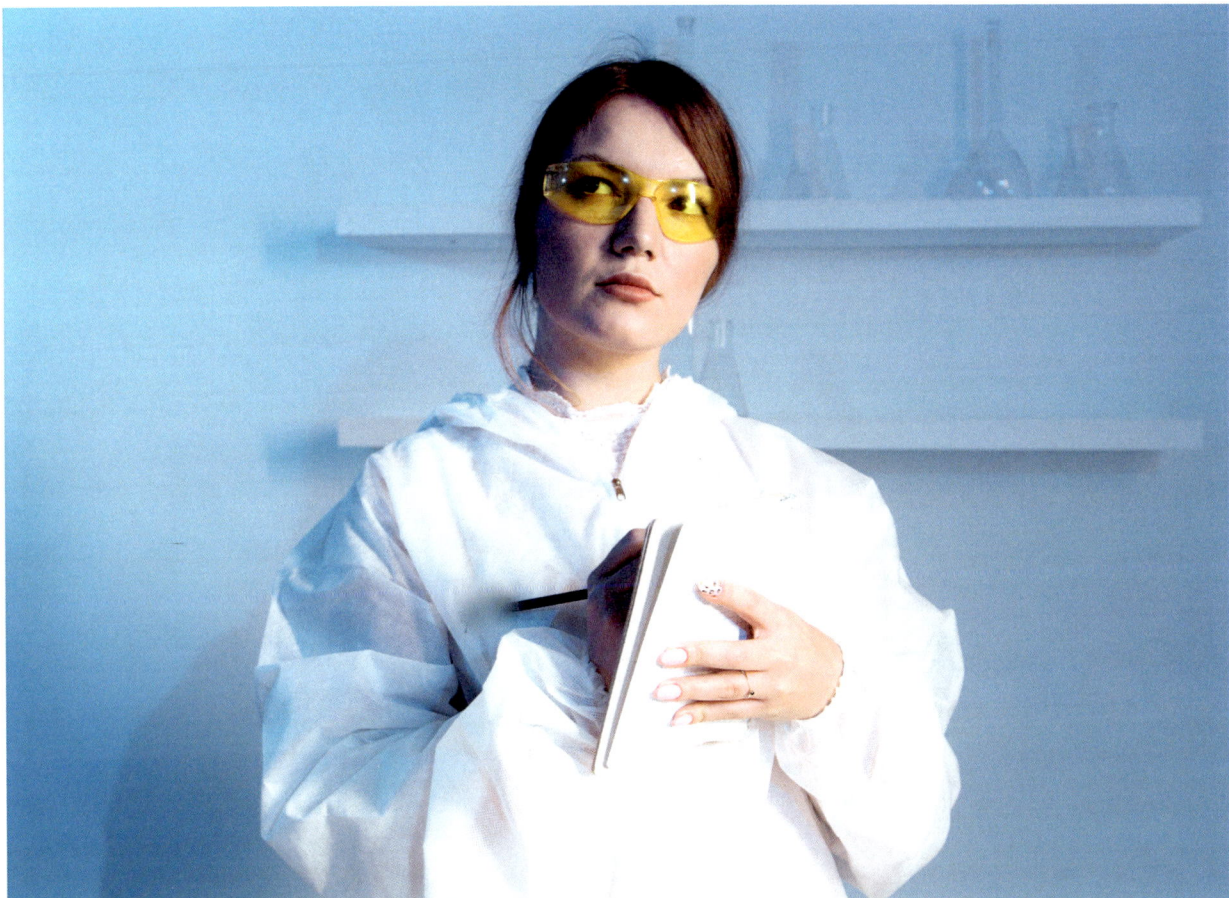

Chapter 12: Conclusion

12.1 The Importance of Knowledge and Skill in Anesthesia Equipment Operation

Throughout this book, we have explored various aspects of anesthesia equipment, including setup, operation, maintenance, troubleshooting, and future trends. It is evident that possessing comprehensive knowledge and skills in anesthesia equipment operation is of paramount importance for anesthesia professionals

12.2 Technological Advancements in Anesthesia Equipment

Anesthesia equipment serves as a critical tool in delivering safe and effective patient care. Understanding the intricacies of different equipment types, their functionalities, and their proper usage is essential for ensuring optimal patient outcomes. By mastering the operation of anesthesia equipment, anesthesia providers and technologists can enhance patient safety, improve efficiency, and contribute to the overall success of anesthesia practice.

12.3 Continuous Learning and Skill Development in Anesthesia

Anesthesia practice is a dynamic field, constantly evolving with new technologies, techniques, and best practices. As anesthesia professionals, it is crucial to embrace a mindset of continuous learning and skill development. By staying updated on the latest advancements, guidelines, and research findings, anesthesia professionals can deliver the highest standard of care to their patients.

Continuous learning encompasses various aspects, including attending educational conferences, participating in workshops, engaging in research activities, and seeking out opportunities for professional development. By actively pursuing continuous learning, anesthesia professionals can enhance their knowledge base, expand their skill set, and adapt to the ever-changing landscape of anesthesia practice.

12.4 Anesthesia Technologists: Fostering a Community of Growth and Learning

Anesthesia technologists play a vital role in anesthesia practice, providing invaluable support to anesthesia providers and contributing to the smooth operation of anesthesia equipment. To further enhance their professional growth, anesthesia technologists are encouraged to actively engage with their peers, share ideas, and ask questions. Fostering a community of growth and learning among anesthesia technologists can propel the field forward and lead to collective advancements.

Collaboration and knowledge sharing among anesthesia technologists can occur through various avenues, such as professional forums, conferences, online communities, and workplace interactions. By sharing experiences, insights, and challenges, anesthesia technologists can learn from each other, gain different perspectives, and collectively contribute to the ongoing improvement of anesthesia practice.

Together, anesthesia providers and technologists form a cohesive team that ensures the safe and effective delivery of anesthesia care. By continuously expanding their knowledge, refining their skills, and fostering a community of growth and learning, anesthesia professionals can elevate the field of anesthesia, improve patient outcomes, and shape the future of anesthesia practice.

In conclusion, the successful operation of anesthesia equipment requires a combination of technical knowledge, practical skills, and a commitment to continuous learning. Anesthesia professionals must embrace the importance of knowledge and skill in equipment operation, continuously update their understanding of emerging trends and advancements, and actively engage in professional development activities. By fostering a community of growth and learning, anesthesia technologists can contribute to the collective advancement of the field and support the anesthesia providers in delivering safe and highquality care. With a dedication to ongoing education and collaboration, anesthesia professionals can navigate the challenges of anesthesia equipment operation and propel the field forward into the future.

12.5 Embracing Innovation and Adapting to Change

In addition to the knowledge and skills discussed in this book, it is crucial for anesthesia professionals to embrace innovation and adapt to the ever-changing landscape of healthcare. The field of anesthesia is constantly evolving, driven by technological advancements, research breakthroughs, and evolving patient needs. To stay at the forefront of anesthesia practice, professionals must be open to new ideas, technologies, and techniques. Embracing innovation allows for the adoption of improved equipment, strategies, and approaches that enhance patient care and outcomes. By staying informed about emerging trends, attending conferences, and engaging in interdisciplinary collaborations, anesthesia professionals can actively contribute to the advancement of the field.

Adapting to change is also essential in the dynamic healthcare environment.

Anesthesia professionals must be flexible and responsive to new regulations, guidelines, and practice standards. This includes incorporating new safety protocols, adjusting workflows to optimize efficiency, and integrating evidencebased practices into daily routines.

12.6 A Call for Collaboration and Communication

Effective communication and collaboration are fundamental to the success of anesthesia practice. Anesthesia professionals must foster an environment of open dialogue, where ideas and concerns can be shared freely. Collaborating with colleagues, including anesthesia providers, technologists, nurses, surgeons, and other healthcare professionals, leads to enhanced patient care, improved outcomes, and a supportive work environment.

By working together, anesthesia professionals can address challenges, share best practices, and learn from one another. Communication extends beyond the immediate team, as anesthesia professionals should also engage in effective patient communication. Clear and empathetic communication with patients ensures their understanding, comfort, and participation in their own care.

12.7 A Journey of Continuous Improvement

Anesthesia equipment operation and patient care are ongoing processes of learning and improvement. As anesthesia professionals embark on their journey, they should remember that excellence is not achieved overnight but through continuous commitment to growth and improvement.

Reflecting on experiences, seeking feedback, and actively seeking opportunities for professional development contribute to this journey.

By striving for continuous improvement, anesthesia professionals can enhance their expertise, optimize patient care, and positively impact the anesthesia community as a whole. This commitment to growth ensures that anesthesia practice remains dynamic, adaptive, and patient-centered.

In Conclusion

Operating anesthesia equipment effectively requires a solid foundation of knowledge, ongoing skill development, and an embrace of innovation and change.

By fostering collaboration, effective communication, and a commitment to continuous improvement, anesthesia professionals can navigate the complexities of their field and provide the highest level of care to their patients.

As anesthesia professionals embark on their careers, they should embrace the importance of ongoing education, adapt to emerging trends, and actively contribute to the advancement of anesthesia practice. By doing so, they will not only enhance their own professional growth but also contribute to the improvement and evolution of anesthesia equipment and patient care.

Through their dedication, anesthesia professionals shape the future of anesthesia practice, ensuring that it remains at the forefront of healthcare and continues to provide safe, efficient, and compassionate care to patients in need.

www.ingramcontent.com/pod-product-compliance
Lightning Source LLC
Chambersburg PA
CBRC090851210326
41597CB00008B/162